ACCESS TO HEALTH CARE IN AMERICA

Committee on Monitoring Access
to Personal Health Care Services

INSTITUTE OF MEDICINE

Michael Millman, Ph.D., *Editor*

NATIONAL ACADEMY PRESS
Washington, D.C.   1993

NATIONAL ACADEMY PRESS • 2101 Constitution Avenue, N.W., Washington, DC 20418

NOTICE: The project that is the subject of this report was approved by the Governing Board of the National Research Council, whose members are drawn from the councils of the National Academy of Sciences, the National Academy of Engineering, and the Institute of Medicine. The members of the committee responsible for the report were chosen for their special competences and with regard for appropriate balance.

This report has been reviewed by a group other than the authors according to procedures approved by a Report Review Committee consisting of members of the National Academy of Sciences, the National Academy of Engineering, and the Institute of Medicine.

The Institute of Medicine was chartered in 1970 by the National Academy of Sciences to enlist distinguished members of the appropriate professions in the examination of policy matters pertaining to the health of the public. In this, the Institute acts under both the Academy's 1863 congressional charter responsibility to be an advisor to the federal government and its own initiative in identifying issues of medical care, research, and education.

This project was supported by the Kellogg Endowment Fund, the Johnson & Johnson Foundation, the Baxter Foundation, the Robert Wood Johnson Foundation (Grant #18455), the Health Care Services Administration (Contract #75-05-0080), Department of Health and Human Services, and Institute of Medicine internal funds.

Library of Congress Cataloging-in-Publication Data

Institute of Medicine (U.S.). Committee on Monitoring Access to
Personal Health Care Services.
    Access to health care in America / Committee on Monitoring Access
to Personal Health Care Services, Institute of Medicine ; Michael
Millman, editor.
       p. cm.
    Includes bibliographical references and index.
    ISBN 0-309-04742-0
    1. Health services accessibility—United States—Evaluation.
I. Millman, Michael L. II. Title.
    [DNLM: 1. Health Services Accessibility—United States. W 76
I592a]
RA407.3.I58   1993
362.1'0973—dc20
DNLM/DLC   92-48299
for Library of Congress   CIP

The serpent has been a symbol of long life, healing, and knowledge among almost all cultures and religions since the beginning of recorded history. The image adopted as a logotype by the Institute of Medicine is based on a relief carving from ancient Greece, now held by the Staatlichemuseen in Berlin.

First Printing, March 1993
Second Printing, February 1994

COMMITTEE ON MONITORING ACCESS TO PERSONAL HEALTH CARE SERVICES

JACK HADLEY (Chair), Co-Director, Georgetown University Center for Health Policy Studies, Washington, D.C.

LU ANN ADAY, Associate Professor of Behavioral Sciences, University of Texas School of Public Health, Houston

JOHN BILLINGS, Health Policy Consultant, New York, New York

CHARLES BRECHER, Professor, New York University, and member, Citizens Budget Commission, Scarsdale, New York

TIMOTHY S. CAREY, Assistant Professor of Medicine, University of North Carolina at Chapel Hill, North Carolina

ALAN B. COHEN, Vice President, The Robert Wood Johnson Foundation, Princeton, New Jersey

EZRA C. DAVIDSON, Jr.,* Professor and Chairman, King/Drew Medical Center, Los Angeles, California

CHESTER W. DOUGLASS, Professor and Chairman, Department of Dental Care Administration, Harvard School of Dental Medicine, Boston, Massachusetts

ARNOLD M. EPSTEIN, Associate Professor of Medicine and Health Care Policy, Harvard University School of Medicine, Boston, Massachusetts

JOHN G. LOEB, Deputy Executive Director, Health Management Corporation, Philadelphia, Pennsylvania

JOANNE E. LUKOMNIK, Special Assistant to the Dean, Albert Einstein College of Medicine, New York, New York

JANET B. MITCHELL, President, Center for Health Economics, Waltham, Massachusetts

IRA MOSCOVICE, Professor and Associate Director, Division of Health Services Research and Policy, University of Minnesota, Minneapolis

DONALD L. PATRICK, Professor, School of Public Health and Community Medicine, University of Washington, Seattle

FERNANDO M. TREVINO, Dean and Professor, School of Health Professions, Southwest Texas State University, San Marcos

GEORGE VAN AMBURG, State Registrar and Chief, Center for Health Statistics, Lansing, Michigan

JOSEPH WESTERMEYER, Professor and Head, Department of Psychiatry and Behavioral Sciences, University of Oklahoma, Oklahoma City

---

*Member, Institute of Medicine

Contents

ACCESS TO
HEALTH CARE
IN
AMERICA

Summary

Beyond the oft-quoted figures about how many Americans are without health insurance, policymakers and the public have few regularly reported indicators to characterize concretely the problems of access to health care services. The images and case stories that appear in the news media give life to the problems of those who cannot obtain the services they need. Yet individual stories cannot systematically reveal the size and changing nature of access problems, their causes, and their effects. The need for this information has been heightened by growing national interest in health care reform, one objective of which is improved access. Whether this objective of federal reform efforts is being achieved cannot be assessed adequately without better health-related indicators.

The mandate of the Institute of Medicine (IOM) to a 17-member committee of experts chosen for the Access Monitoring Project was to develop a set of indicators for monitoring access to personal health care services at the national level over time. It was envisioned that these indicators would be akin to national economic indicators—the unemployment rate, new housing starts, the inflation rate, consumer confidence surveys—which provide a picture of the state of the economy and how it might be changing. Similarly, access indicators would allow us to track whether conditions for obtaining care, particularly among vulnerable groups in society, were improving or getting worse. In addition, like economic indicators, the expectation of routinely available reports would stimulate national debate about needed policy actions and the consequences of actions taken.

The focus of this report, like the committee's deliberations, is on access to personal health services—the one-on-one interaction of provider and patient. The committee chose five objectives of personal health care to organize its indicators: successful birth outcomes, reducing the incidence of preventable diseases, early detection and diagnosis of treatable diseases, reducing the effect of chronic diseases and prolonging life, and reducing morbidity and pain through timely and appropriate treatment. This specific focus on personal health care does not gainsay the important investments society can make in population-based strategies in such areas as the environment, pollutants, health education, occupational health, and injury control. Policies in these fields could potentially save more lives and have a greater impact on quality of life than programs to extend health services. Nonetheless, the large proportion of the nation's resources being devoted to personal health care has provoked considerable interest in monitoring those investments from the standpoint of equity of access.

The IOM committee's approach to developing indicators was to find measures that would track the use of services known to have measurable effects—for example, prenatal care. An outcome of using these effective services—fewer low-birthweight infants—is also an indicator of access to services that can be monitored. Analysis of these indicators would provide information on the effects of health policies; the data could be used in turn in making choices with regard to the three major concerns of health care policymaking: access, quality, and cost.

This study had two key objectives: first, to propose an initial set of indicators that lays the groundwork for the evolution of a monitoring system and, second, to use those indicators to assess the current state of access at the national level. The first objective entailed clarifying what is really meant by saying we want to improve access and translating concerns about who cannot get what type of care into a limited and cohesive set of indicators that can offer reliable and valid measurements. Applying these indicators to produce an assessment about access, the second objective, involved obtaining a decade's worth of data, analyzing the data, and interpreting the meaning of trends.

Although the state of the art of monitoring access is still at an elementary stage, there is sufficient information available to draw some important conclusions. In most instances the basic data bases exist to measure the indicators chosen, but crucial modifications in how and when data are collected are necessary to make them more useful for monitoring. The committee offers numerous recommendations in this report for the data collection and research needed to push the evolution of monitoring forward at a faster, surer pace.

GENERAL CONCLUSIONS ON THE STATE OF ACCESS

As a whole, indicators of access to personal health care services provide little encouraging evidence of progress over the past decade. Stagnation is the single best word to characterize our current state. Successes like improvements in breast cancer screening are counterbalanced by the return of diseases that can be avoided, like tuberculosis and congenital syphilis. Underlying most of the indicators is a growing division between the haves and the have-nots in our society.

A large group of citizens in this country make contact with medical providers only a little more than half as often as their fellows. This group lacks health care coverage and is generally at the low end of the income scale. Indicators that measure health outcomes suggest that at least for people from low-income neighborhoods the difference in health care use has a profound impact on their health and well-being. Admission rates to hospitals for conditions that should be controlled with appropriate ambulatory care are on average four times higher for residents of low-income than for high-income neighborhoods. The committee believes that evidence is building to demonstrate that no or inadequate health care coverage is the reason many of these people fail to obtain the timely and appropriate care that would make a difference in the state of their health. Further work is required, however, to establish solid causal linkages between the access barriers of lack of health insurance, low income, and nonfinancial factors such as culture and geographic isolation and measures of outcome such as premature death, sickness, disability, and avoidable hospitalization.

Compared with other groups in society, blacks and some ethnic minorities are more likely to have low incomes and inadequate health insurance. The effects of these burdens are borne out by utilization and outcome indicators virtually across the board. There is evidence of inequity in the timely receipt of ambulatory care, immunizations, dental visits, and some sophisticated procedures. Even in instances in which general improvement can be seen that spans the U.S. population, improvement is slower for these groups—especially blacks.

Some of the most striking differences can be found in mortality rates by race. After controlling for a number of behavioral risk factors, a wide gap persists between mortality rates of middle-aged black men and women and their white counterparts. A reasonable estimate is that one-third to one-half of the gap may be attributable to access problems. In 1970 black infants were 85 percent more likely than whites to die during the first year of life; by 1988 black infants were more than twice as likely as whites to die during their first year. A related measure is the slow but steadily growing disparity in low birthweights for blacks and whites during the past 20 years.

DEFINING ACCESS

Access is a shorthand term for a broad set of concerns that center on the degree to which individuals and groups are able to obtain needed services from the medical care system. Often because of difficulties in defining and measuring the concept, people equate access with insurance coverage or with having enough doctors and hospitals in the geographic area in which they live. But having insurance or nearby health care providers is no guarantee that people who need services will get them. Conversely, many who lack coverage or live in areas that appear to have shortages of health care resources do, indeed, receive services.

For the purposes of its work the committee defined access as follows: **the timely use of personal health services to achieve the best possible health outcomes.** An important characteristic of this definition is that it relies on both the use of health services and health outcomes as yardsticks for judging whether access has been achieved. The test of **equity** of access involves determining whether there are systematic differences in use and outcomes among groups in U.S. society and whether these differences result from financial or other barriers to care.

In applying its definition of access, the committee sought to occupy a practical middle ground between all care that people might want or need and the belief that medical care can make an important difference in people's lives. The definition forces us to identify those areas of medical care in which services can be shown to influence health status and then to ask whether the relatively poorer outcomes of some population groups can be explained by problems related to access. The definition also emphasizes the need to move beyond standard approaches that rely mainly on enumerating health care providers, the uninsured, or encounters with health care providers to detect access problems.

No matter how generally efficacious a particular health service may be, a good health outcome cannot always be guaranteed. The most important consideration is whether people have the opportunity for a good outcome—especially in those instances in which medical care can make a difference. When those opportunities are systematically denied to groups in society, there is an access problem that needs to be addressed.

The access monitoring indicators recommended by the committee are intended to detect when and where access problems occur in the personal health care system. They do not explain the exact causes of these problems, but they can provide a better basis for generating theories about why differences in access exist among populations. Although they are only proxies for complicated phenomena, over time the indicators give important information about the direction and speed of change. They also provide clues about the relative status of groups of people at the same moment in time. Indicators will not always move in the same direction. Some may increase, some may decline, and others may show no change. Although this makes overall assessments more complicated, it can be useful to highlight problems and gains in specific areas.

The committee focused on access problems that it believed, if corrected, were most likely to lead to improved health outcomes across the age spectrum. It identified indicators that could be used to measure changes in the degree of access to specific types of personal health care (defined as the one-on-one interaction of provider and patient). The committee's deliberations resulted in a list of 15 indicators that were grouped into several distinct categories. These categories define a set of national objectives (see above) for the personal health care system; each set of indicators provides a means for assessing progress toward a specific objective.

THE COMMITTEE'S INDICATORS AND PROGRESS TOWARD ACCESS OBJECTIVES

Objective 1: Promoting Successful Birth Outcomes

Numerous studies have shown links between the early initiation, amount, and content of prenatal care and birth outcomes. Outcomes that indicate problems in access include infant mortality, low birthweight, and incidence of congenital syphilis.

For all races slightly less than 70 percent of all women received adequate prenatal care in each year from 1986 to 1988. The percentage of women receiving early care increased steadily during the 1970s (from 67.9 percent for all races in 1970 to 75.9 percent in 1979) but remained static between 1980 and 1988. There is a striking difference between whites and blacks in receiving adequate prenatal care (73.5 and 50.7 percent, respectively) (Figure 1).

The U.S. infant mortality rate dropped 7 percentage points between 1989 and 1990, a significantly greater decline than occurred during previous years of the decade when the average annual decline was less than 3 percentage points. The average rate of decline during the 1980s was well below the annual average of 4.7 percentage points. However, the greatest portion of the decrease during the past two decades was in neonatal deaths, which probably reflects improvements in medical technology rather than better prenatal care. With respect to low birthweight, some decline in rates occurred during the 1970s, but no improvement was apparent during the 1980s.

Each case of congenital syphilis indicates either a lack of any prenatal care (even one prenatal care visit should alert a health care provider to the need for treatment) or a lack of adequate care (a prenatal visit at which an infected mother is not diagnosed is inadequate). Treatment of syphilis at least 30 days prior to delivery should prevent infection in the infant.

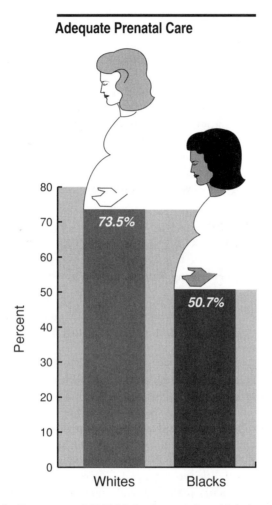

Adequate Prenatal Care

FIGURE 1   Percentage of 1988 births, by race, for which the mother received what is considered adequate prenatal care. The data on which this figure is based come from 49 states and the District of Columbia, as reported by the National Center for Health Statistics.

The recent rise in U.S. congenital syphilis rates—they tripled from 1989 to 1990 (Figure 2)—is thought to be due in part to the increase in cocaine use (particularly "crack" cocaine), with its attendant transmission of sexually transmitted diseases. Rates of congenital syphilis therefore may also indicate a lack of available, acceptable, and effective drug treatment services for pregnant women.

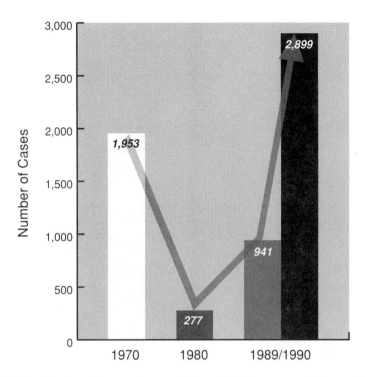

Congenital Syphilis

FIGURE 2 Number of cases of congenital syphilis (i.e., among infants up to age 1) for selected years, according to data from the Centers for Disease Control.

Objective 2: Reducing the Incidence of Vaccine-Preventable Childhood Diseases

There are few instances in which personal health care can virtually prevent a disease from occurring. Access to immunization for childhood diseases provides the best current example of this potential of health care services. Figure 3 shows that less than half of nonwhite preschoolers in 1985 were immunized for measles and less than two-thirds of white pre-schoolers were so immunized.

Although surveys of immunization have been infrequent and plagued with methodological problems, those that have been conducted indicate declines since 1970 in the vaccination levels for diphtheria-pertussis-tetanus (DPT) and polio for preschool children. There are no clear trends in the

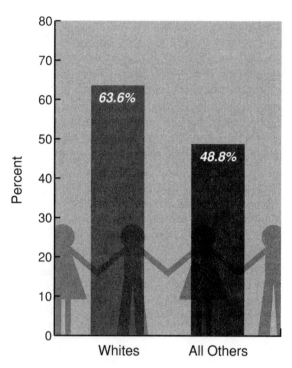

Preschool Immunization for Measles

FIGURE 3   Percentage of preschool (children ages 1–4) immunizations for measles in 1985 for whites and all other ethnic groups.   This figure is based on data from the U.S. Immunization Survey, conducted by the Centers for Disease Control.

vaccination rates for other diseases, particularly during 1983–1985.   Because disease occurrence is cyclical in nature, caution must be exercised in interpreting trends from year to year.   Nonetheless, in theory no child should contract these diseases if most are immunized.   Recent outbreaks of measles and DPT are particularly disturbing sentinel events in this regard.

Objective 3:   Early Detection and Diagnosis of Treatable Diseases

There are a number of diseases for which early detection is important enough to justify screening large segments of the population.   For screening to be worthwhile, an effective medical intervention must be available for treating the disease of interest at an early stage.   The committee focused on screening for breast and cervical cancer.   Although public health education efforts are critical for creating awareness of screening tests, the personal health care system must ensure that providers follow through with periodic testing and provide appropriate treatment when disease is identified.

As of 1987 only about two-thirds of U.S. women over the age of 18 had had a Pap smear in the previous three years to detect cervical cancer. Hispanic women are less likely to have had the procedure than black or white women. In addition to problems of access to these services for minority women in general, the elderly are of special concern. Elderly white women were more than twice as likely as younger white women never to have had the procedure (22.6 percent of elderly white women had not had the test). About twice this proportion (43 percent) of older minority women reported never having had a Pap smear. Figure 4 shows the percentages of women who have never had a Pap smear.

Recent studies seem to indicate a dramatic increase in mammography

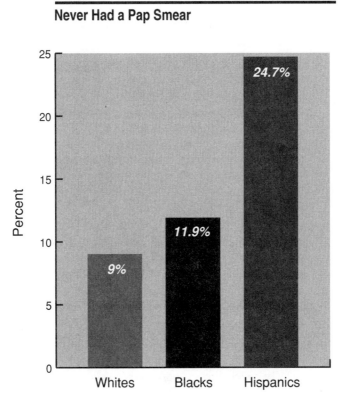

Never Had a Pap Smear

FIGURE 4 Percentage of white, black, and Hispanic women in 1987 who were 18 years of age and older and had never had a Pap smear. The percentages were derived from National Health Interview Survey data for 1987.

Mammograms

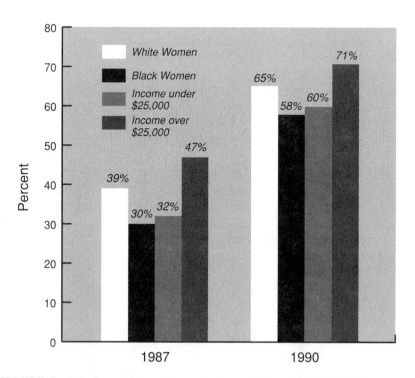

FIGURE 5   This figure shows changes between 1987 and 1990 in (1) the percentages of black and white women age 40 and older who reported ever having had a
mammogram and (2) the percentages of women of that age reporting mammography
who had incomes over $25,000 and under $25,000. The 1987 percentages are based
on data from the National Health Interview Survey of that year; the 1990 percentages were calculated from data collected by the Mammography Attitudes and Usage
Study conducted by the Jacobs Institute of Women's Health with technical assistance from the National Cancer Institute.

screening, although differences persist by age, race, and income (Figure 5).
Mammogram screening increased between 1987 and 1990 probably as a
result of media coverage and enhanced public health promotion efforts. By
1990, among women over age 40, 64 percent reported having ever had a
mammogram, nearly twice the proportion reporting mammography three
years earlier.

   The progression of cancer can occur despite appropriate therapy, but
discovery of late-stage cancers may also indicate underuse of an effective

screening test. Alternatively, or in addition, late-stage cancer may also reflect inappropriate medical follow-up of a diagnosed disease. Either or both of these explanations may apply to findings showing that individuals living in high-income areas had about 10 percent fewer cases of late-stage breast cancers in the mid-1980s compared with an earlier time period in the mid-1970s. Low-income areas improved only about half as much over the same time period.

Among whites the proportion of cases of late-stage cervical cancer remained approximately the same in the 1970s and 1980s. In contrast, the proportion of late-stage diagnoses for blacks, which had been approximately the same as for whites in the mid-1970s, nearly doubled by the mid-1980s. With respect to income levels, only a small difference persists over time, and that gap appears to be narrowing.

Objective 4: Reducing the Effects of Chronic Disease and Prolonging Life

Many of the reasons people use medical care are related to the treatment of chronic conditions. These diseases usually are not self-limiting but are ongoing over an extended period of time. Adverse consequences of chronic conditions can occur with or without regular medical care, but negative consequences are more common when regular care is absent. Even when life cannot be extended, health care can contribute to improved functioning for individuals with chronic disease and can minimize discomfort. The committee chose to track chronic disease follow-up care by examining patterns of physician use and use of high-cost discretionary procedures. The two outcome indicators focus on states of illness that require hospital admission and an experimental measure of access-related excess mortality to detect racial differences (described above in the general conclusions).

Having health care coverage makes a major difference in whether people who believe themselves to be in poor health have at least one physician contact within a year. In 1989 the uninsured were more than twice as likely to go without physician contact as those with private health insurance, Medicaid, or Medicare. Figure 6 shows the proportion of persons with no physician visits in the past year, among those who rated themselves as being in poor or fair health in 1989 (the committee's indirect indicator of an underlying chronic disease).

As an indicator, referral-sensitive surgeries reach beyond entry into the personal health care system to assess a second level of access—expensive discretionary procedures. That this is a problem worth monitoring emerges from the medical literature, which contains examples of medical and surgical procedures for which there are differences in utilization according to patient health insurance status, race, and other sociodemographic factors. If

Poor or Fair Health and No Physician Visits

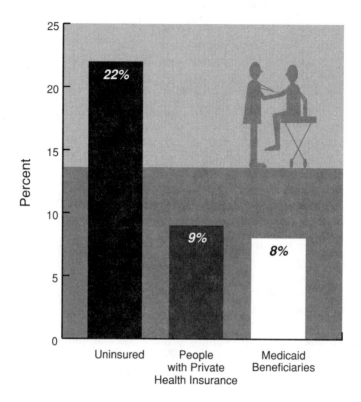

FIGURE 6   Percentage of people in 1989 who were in poor or fair health (by their own report) and who did not contact a physician. The figure, which is based on data from the 1989 National Health Interview Survey, shows the percentages by health insurance status.

one considers ratios of low-income to high-income area admission rates for all referral-sensitive procedures combined, people from poor areas appear to be about two-thirds as likely to obtain the services. The most marked differences in rates of use of procedures were for breast reconstruction, coronary artery bypass grafts, and coronary angiography.

Ongoing medical management can effectively control the severity and progression of a number of chronic diseases, even if the diseases themselves cannot be prevented. An advanced stage of a chronic disease requiring hospitalization may indicate the existence of one or more access barriers to personal health care services. Thus, hospital admissions for certain

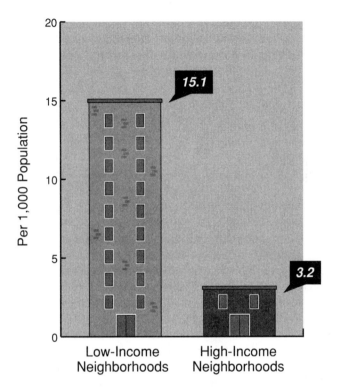

Hospital Admissions for Chronic Conditions

FIGURE 7 Number of hospital admissions for relatively controllable chronic conditions per 1,000 people from low- and high-income neighborhoods. (The low- and high-income designations were developed by using zip codes and Census Bureau information.) The figures are a joint product of the Codman Research Group, the Ambulatory Care Access Project (United Hospital Fund of New York), and the IOM Access Monitoring Committee.

conditions are a potentially useful indicator of the performance of the ambulatory health care system. High rates of admissions for conditions related to treatable chronic diseases, in particular, may provide indirect evidence of serious patient access problems or deficiencies in outpatient management (see Figure 7).

In comparisons of hospital admission rates for people from low- and high-income zip codes, all of the ambulatory-care-sensitive admission rates were substantially higher for low-income areas. The overall average ratio was 4.65. The greatest differences—ranging from six- to sevenfold—were related to admissions for congestive heart failure, hypertension, and asthma. Yet even the lowest ratio, for the diagnosis of angina, showed income differences almost threefold in magnitude.

Objective 5: Reducing Morbidity and Pain
Through Timely and Appropriate Treatment

The primary medical concern of the 90 percent of people who see themselves as being in good health is, Will I be able to see a doctor if I become sick? One utilization indicator for this objective attempts to measure this concern by singling out healthy people who suddenly become so sick that they must reduce their normal activities. The question is whether such characteristics as insurance status, income, and race have an effect on whether medical attention is obtained. A related outcome indicator looks at the effects of delayed or inappropriate outpatient treatment for acute disease by relying on analysis of admission rates by zip code for a select group of diagnoses.

A second utilization indicator moves from medical care to dental care, a set of services that have limited insurance coverage and thus the potential for being highly income sensitive. Dental services also represent an area of personal health care in which treatment, although usually not life saving, contributes to general well-being and social functioning.

People without insurance and Medicare recipients without supplementary policies were more likely than those with private insurance to refrain from seeking medical care or advice when sick. The differences for both groups compared with those with private insurance are about 10 percentage points. The likelihood of contacting a physician decreases by about 5 percentage points at the lowest income levels for the uninsured and the privately insured. Presumably, anticipated out-of-pocket costs are deterring some of the insured from obtaining services.

People who see themselves as being in good to excellent health—the population of interest in this objective—may seek medical attention for any number of reasons. The personal health care system in some cases provides only symptomatic relief to patients for conditions that would resolve independent of any medical intervention. In other situations, however, symptoms that are not addressed in a timely fashion can evolve into acute medical problems requiring hospitalization. Mild cases of such infections as bacterial pneumonia, cellulitis, kidney diseases, and precursor conditions leading to pelvic inflammatory disease can often be managed with antibiotics in outpatient settings, preventing the disease from becoming more severe. For most of the diagnoses used in this indicator, admissions from low-income zip codes were two to five times higher than admissions from high-income zip codes.

Annual Dental Care

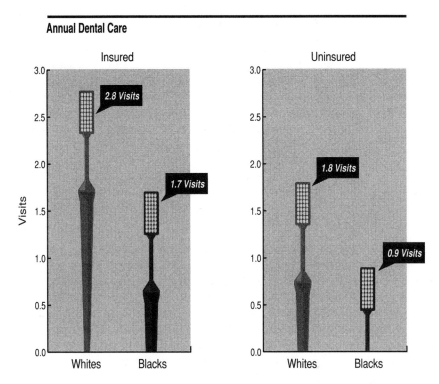

FIGURE 8 Number of annual dental visits by whites and blacks (according to data from the 1989 National Health Interview Survey) for those with and without private insurance.

In general, the use of dental care has been increasing, but there are serious inequities in use based on insurance, race, and income differences. Between 1983 and 1989 the number of dental visits per person in the United States increased 17 percent, from 1.8 to 2.1. During the same period the proportion of those who had never visited a dentist fell from 7.7 percent to 6.4 percent.

In 1989 those with dental insurance made an average of about one more visit to the dentist than those without insurance (2.7 in comparison to 1.7). Consistent differences between whites and blacks persisted despite insurance coverage (Figure 8). As income increases, the difference between the number of visits by those with insurance and those without decreases.

RECOMMENDATIONS

A major aim of the IOM Access Monitoring Project was to improve the state of the art in measuring access problems by determining what indicators can be identified now, what important access problems do not have indicators, and what steps need to be taken over the long term to institutionalize a monitoring system based on valid, reliable data. The purpose of these activities was to create a basis by which decisionmakers could determine how the nation is faring with respect to access over time. Toward this end, the committee has formulated a set of recommendations arising out of its general review of the indicators, trends in the data, and problems in measurement and methodology encountered in the course of its analyses. By way of summary, some overarching themes from the recommendations are worth highlighting.

• *Federal Role*   The committee recommends that there be a federal organization responsible for monitoring access to personal health services. This ongoing function should include the central collection, analysis, improvement, and dissemination of information on changes in access. The same organization should have the responsibility to provide technical assistance and consultation to local organizations that conduct their own analyses of access indicators. These efforts should include activities to encourage improved technical capacity and to promote, where appropriate, consistent definitions and analytic approaches.

• *State and Local Monitoring*   States and local communities would benefit from a national access monitoring process. At the national level, the utilization and outcome indicators selected for this report are intended to be sensitive to the direction and extent of change in structural, financial, and personal barriers. At the state and local levels, these barriers are increasingly definable in terms of a specific set of Medicaid benefits, institutional providers, population demographics, and physical features of the environment. Thus, the advantage of proximity is being able to relate changes to more concrete circumstances. The problem is that either local data are incomplete or there are insufficient resources to analyze the local data that do exist. To address this problem, it is necessary first to identify clearly what data are needed (i.e., develop a monitoring framework) and how the data might be interpreted; a cost-effective strategy for obtaining missing data should then be devised and implemented.

The committee has proposed a framework for monitoring access and has analyzed specific indicators, demonstrating how they might be related to barriers. As a first step, in areas for which local data are available, states and localities can compare themselves with the national averages. They can also use additional data (e.g., from surveys intended to determine which physicians accept Medicaid) and their general familiarity with the contours of the local health care system—knowledge that is not available at the national level—to draw conclusions about access problems faced by their vulnerable populations. In addition, decisions about whether to invest in new data collection can be helped by the knowledge of what can be done with the data. Understanding the potential payoffs, and the extent to which emerging national trends apply to local circumstances, will allow communities to determine their data collection needs.

The committee recognizes that constrained state and local public health budgets are likely to limit investments in major new surveys, hospital discharge data collection systems, and cancer registries. To the extent that upfront research and development costs can be borne by the federal government or foundations, the cost of implementing enhanced data systems could be reduced for local jurisdictions.

• *Racial and Ethnic Differences*   Anyone who reads this report will be struck by the persistent and in some cases widening disparities in access between blacks and whites. Studies of health care access that compare the experience of whites with that of racial and ethnic minorities other than blacks frequently reveal similar disparities. When certain factors, such as insurance status and income, are taken into account, some of these disparities diminish. There continues to be a need to oversample minorities in national surveys as well as to conduct specialized surveys focused on minorities. To understand the roles that income and insurance play, all surveys should include questions that elicit such information.

Because it is not always feasible to improve the utility of national data bases—that is, by recording the race or ethnicity of patients—it will be necessary to mount studies that more fully characterize unexplained problems of access.

• *Directions for Health Services Research*   In its analysis the committee has reaffirmed that lack of health care coverage is, to a great extent, a good proxy for access. Evidence is mounting about the role insurance plays in influencing not only health care use but outcomes as well. Much work remains to be done in fleshing out these relationships.

Nonetheless, the committee is convinced that other factors play an important role in explaining differences in access to care. This sense is illustrated by the experience of other industrialized nations in which financial barriers to services have been removed but serious inequities among various population groups still occur. Many believe that these inequities would be diminished by changes in the way the delivery of care is organized and by greater responsiveness of providers to the personal and cultural characteristics of their clients. Thus, the committee has concluded that, even if the United States were to adopt universal entitlement, achieving the objectives around which its indicators are organized is likely to remain a great challenge. Further research into these aspects of access is clearly needed.

The limitations of confining measures of equity of access to financial variables are nowhere better illustrated than by those health services that must be combined with effective social services and public health planning for good results. Good prenatal care, for example, must be concerned with how the nutritional needs of the pregnant woman will be met. This service-integration feature, generally acknowledged for prenatal care, is also present in a set of topics that the committee identified for further development as access indicators. These topics represent access problems that may be amenable to solutions requiring close linkages among personal health care services, public health, and social services. In other words, the access problems of homeless people, migrants, people with disabilities, patients with the acquired immune deficiency syndrome (AIDS), and victims of domestic violence will not be solved with an insurance card alone. The complexity of the problems these people face taxes our current understanding of how to measure access barriers. Their problems require organizational solutions that include continuity of care, integration of services, and other subtle characteristics. Tracking these access problems will require measurement skills and methodologies that lie beyond our current capabilities.

1

Introduction

Most Americans find it difficult to reconcile their notions of social justice with the fact that some 35 million people, most of whom are employed or are dependents of someone employed, lack basic health insurance coverage. We hear that government agencies, physicians, and public and private hospitals are straining to keep pace with requests for services amid budget constraints. Not only are some people losing their insurance coverage, but the size of vulnerable populations is growing. Progress against several health problems is blocked because of poor access to health care. The news media frequently depict the plight of poor unwed pregnant adolescents, children in low-income families, the homeless, minority groups, residents of rural areas, and refugees. When the focus shifts to whether we are making headway against specific diseases, the disparity in health status between vulnerable groups and the general populace becomes apparent. With respect to HIV/AIDS, drug abuse, cancer, and infant mortality, less favorable outcomes are often attributed to the inability of some segments of society to gain timely access to essential health services.

In addition to concerns over the less fortunate in our society, there is a growing uneasiness that the delivery system and insurance infrastructure are not meeting the needs of middle- and upper-income Americans as well as they once were. Many besides the poor may have difficulty getting access to health care. Those with preexisting disease conditions fear that they will lose insurance coverage if they change jobs. Middle-income people fear that shrinking insurance benefits will force them to pay more and more of the costs of health care, increasing their reluctance to seek care when they need it. Spurred in part by the malpractice insurance crisis, obstetrical services are reported to be in short supply in some areas. Residents of this country's rural areas are fighting an uphill battle to keep hospitals open so that, at a minimum, they have access to emergency services and essential primary care. To avoid having to admit emergency room patients who may not have insurance, growing numbers of hospitals have ceased offering emergency services.

There is no shortage of stories depicting these and related problems. What policymakers and the public lack, however, is a systematic way of looking at the barriers people face in getting needed health care and the impact those barriers have on society. Data describing barriers to health care are incomplete, scattered, underanalyzed, or outdated. The information that has been gathered is not organized in ways that promote systematic thinking about how access to health care has changed over time, nor can differences among affected groups be compared. For these and other reasons, the desirable objective of improving access to health care remains elusive.

The IOM Access Monitoring Project was designed to develop a way to monitor access to health care that will be useful to health care policymakers. The charge to the IOM committee was to develop a rationale and framework for gauging how well or how poorly the nation provides access to personal health care. The focus of this effort was to be the development of a limited set of indicators that could reliably sense the direction and extent of change at the national level in access problems and at the same time give clues about what factors might be driving that change. In addition to clarifying perceptions about the status of health care access in the United States, it was hoped that these indicators would serve as a general guide to decisionmaking.

Unfortunately, the data and methods available to devise a reliable system for monitoring access to health care are incomplete in some areas. Thus, in addition to developing indicators, the committee was instructed to recommend strategies for improving state-of-the-art access monitoring. This included identifying ways to enhance ongoing data collection activities and refine measurement techniques as well as encouraging research on access problems in areas in which there are currently insufficient data or in which the appropriate indicator for measuring access is unclear.

BACKGROUND

Unlike many of IOM's activities, this project was self-initiated—neither mandated by federal legislation nor directly requested by a public or private agency. The call for such a study of health care access came from the IOM membership, and the specific direction taken was one that emerged from meetings of IOM's Board on Health Care Services.

The board concluded that, because of both societal changes and shifts in public policy, better mechanisms are required for monitoring changes in access. The nation needs, but currently lacks, an entity to continuously monitor the numerous types of utilization and health status problems arising from insurance inadequacies, cultural impediments, geographic barriers, or other factors and place these problems in the broader context of national health policies. The 14-member IOM access monitoring committee was constituted in February 1990 as a first step toward this goal.

Although the mandate for this specific project was generated by the interest of IOM members, the idea to undertake a monitoring project had its intellectual roots in a 1985 workshop sponsored by IOM. In fact, many of the indicators discussed at that meeting, as well as the workshop's conclusion that access monitoring should focus on health care utilization, were incorporated into the present committee's work.

The 1985 workshop was the result of discussions among IOM, the Robert Wood Johnson Foundation, and the federal Health Resources and Services Administration, which was seeking better methods for targeting its dollars to the medically underserved. In its 1985 annual report the foundation's then-president David Rogers expressed the frustrations that led to the workshop:

> Each day a quick glance at the newspaper tells us the relative standing of our baseball, football, and ice hockey teams. Likewise, a myriad of data is available daily on the status of American business or the economy in our major cities. Yet in health care, even fairly simple statistics are not regularly collected, or when they are, they are processed so slowly that they are not available until two to five years after the fact. (Rogers, 1985)

DEVELOPING A SET OF INDICATORS

The process of developing social indicators involves in principle at least three broad elements (DeNeufville, 1975). First, the concepts that underlie the phenomenon of interest—access, in this case—need to be made clear with the help of existing models and attempts at problem definition. Second, the constraints on and possibilities for quantifying the concepts with existing or new data need to be considered. Third, it must be determined how best to organize and summarize the data so that they are of most use to policymakers.

The development of IOM's access monitoring framework and set of specific indicators was an interactive process. The committee initially identified an extensive list of indicators that it believed to be both broadly representative of access problems and for which there was a possibility of regularly available information. Each meeting of the committee was followed by study of the methodological issues and assessment of data availability related to individual indicators. The indicator list and the conceptual framework were then refined at each subsequent meeting. When gaps in the information base were found, the committee recommended ways to fill those gaps. Many of the recommendations were directed at public and private organizations that collect information intended to enhance the nation's ability to monitor access to personal health care services. Taken together, the recommendations constitute a research agenda.

The committee also identified a second set of potential indicators representative of important access problems but for which a lack of data or consensus about how they should be measured limited the degree to which they could be studied. Descriptions of these access problems are included in Chapter 3. It is the committee's belief that further studies in these areas are an important component of a research agenda. To begin the process of moving toward developing these indicators, the committee commissioned three background papers on AIDS, substance abuse, and migrants and people who are homeless (Appendixes A–C). The papers identify what is needed to develop useful indicators and other approaches that may be used for tracking access problems.

RELATIONSHIP OF ACCESS MONITORING TO OTHER RELEVANT ACTIVITIES

The aim of the IOM Access Monitoring Project was to improve the state of the art in measuring access problems by determining what indicators can be identified now, what important access problems do not have indicators, and what steps need to be taken over the long term to institutionalize a monitoring system based on valid, reliable data. The purpose of these activities is to create a data base that will allow decisionmakers to determine how the nation is faring with respect to access over time. The data base should allow both general assessments of access to health care in the United States and specific analyses of particular services or populations.

It is expected that evidence of time-dependent changes in access, and differences in access among population groups, will stimulate focused discussion about policies that can promote more appropriate utilization and better health outcomes. Although the indicators may suggest how well or how poorly current policies are working, the IOM monitoring project is not an evaluation study per se. A specific change in Medicaid eligibility, for example, cannot be detected by and ascribed to changes in one or more indicators because many other policies and forces are operating at the same time. In the future, however, evaluators may want to use the indicators as part of studies that take into account other factors that may explain changes in access.

Although the monitoring project is not a research effort, the committee has relied heavily on the studies of others. Particular attention has been devoted to research that examines services known to affect health status, the independent contribution of barriers to use, and health outcomes. This report includes some original analyses of survey and hospital discharge data to demonstrate the utility of specific types of analyses; it was not feasible, however, to pursue inquiries into all the lines of interest. It is hoped that this report will spark interest in focused research in a variety of areas.

The IOM Access Monitoring Project overlaps with several other efforts to develop health indicators, most notably the Year 2000 Health Objectives for the Nation, outlined in *Healthy People* (U.S. Department of Health and Human Services, 1991). These objectives focus principally on health promotion and protection and on preventive health services. Several of the IOM indicators fall within these categories. Where there is overlap, the IOM committee has attempted to be as consistent as possible with the Year 2000 Health Objectives, which serve as useful standards to assess how far the nation might be from access goals. The main focus of the IOM project, however, is personal health services, including curative medical services. Other factors that can affect health and that are addressed in *Healthy People*, such as traffic accidents, misuse of firearms, environmental controls, and safe work environments, are not dealt with by the IOM project. In contrast to the great breadth of *Healthy People*, other monitoring projects have focused on particular subpopulations, particularly children and pregnant women.

Additionally, the World Health Organization (1981) has developed a set of indicators as part of its Health for All Project. Although the WHO literature offers some useful ideas (particularly in the area of avoidable mortality), many of the indicators are broad social and economic measures (e.g., income distribution, adult literacy rate) rather than specifically health-related gauges or are not germane to the U.S. context (e.g., distance to protected clean water supply, malaria prophylaxis).

MAJOR DATA SOURCES: THEIR USES AND LIMITATIONS

Box 1-1 shows the major sources of data on which the committee drew to support the monitoring of access indicators. The sources cover a wide array of activities designed to measure different types of health services use and health states. Each data base has inherent strengths and weaknesses, and, although they hold great promise for access measurement, none were established with this as a principal or even secondary aim in mind. Therefore, the major challenge for the future will be to capitalize on their strengths while making the necessary changes to minimize the weaknesses that limit our ability to draw conclusions from available data about access problems. These changes must be judicious so as not to interfere with the original

BOX 1-1 Major Data Sources for Monitoring
Access to Personal Health Care

Data Type	Data Sources	Sponsoring Agencies
Vital statistics	Birth certificate Death certificate	National Center for Health Statistics (compiled from state data)
Surveys	National Health Interview Survey	National Center for Health Statistics
Complementary	National Medical Expenditure Survey	Agency for Health Care Policy and Research
	Current Beneficiary Survey (Medicare)	Health Care Financing Administration
	Access surveys	The Robert Wood Johnson Foundation
	National Maternal and Infant Health Survey	National Center for Health Statistics
	Behavioral Risk Factor Survey	Centers for Disease Control
	Mortality Followback Survey	National Center for Health Statistics
Examination	National Health and Nutrition Examination Survey (NHANES) (Epidemiological followback surveys; Hispanic HANES)	National Center for Health Statistics
Hospital discharge data	State hospital discharge data bases	Approximately 24 states
Notifiable diseases	Provider case- occurrence reports	Collected by the Centers for Disease Control from 52 areas in the U.S. and five territories
Disease registries	State and local cancer registries	Compiled by the National Cancer Institute

purposes of the data collection activities. How to approach this challenge is a major focus of the committee's recommendations on ways to improve the state of the art of access monitoring.

Strengths and Weaknesses

Vital Statistics

Vital statistics are derived from birth and death certificates. The birth certificate is the major source of information about the use of prenatal care and low birthweight. In general, physician records about a woman's visits during pregnancy are transferred to the hospital for inclusion on the certificate. However, information on a birth record about the content of prenatal visits is limited. Data problems arise either when women have no or multiple providers or when recall of service use is required after delivery. Thus, threats to the validity of the data come from those most likely to have poor pregnancy outcomes—the poor, the young, minorities, noncitizens illegally residing in the United States, and the poorly educated.

Death records provide mortality statistics and when linked to the birth record offer insight into the important correlates of infant mortality related to prenatal care. The cause-of-death information recorded on a death certificate can be used to compare the mortality experience of different subpopulations and to assess its relationship to access barriers. Concerns have been expressed about the accuracy of cause-of-death information because it is based on the judgment of the certifying physician.

For the purposes of monitoring access for all age groups, the major limitation of the death certificate is its lack of relevant information on the possible extent of access barriers as a result of lack of insurance, low income, or other such impediments. This limitation can be overcome in part through special followback surveys of a patient's closest relative.

Surveys

Large household surveys such as the National Health Interview Survey (NHIS) provide a wealth of information that allows analysts to relate the use of health services and self-reports of health status to characteristics of individuals and families. Key strengths of the NHIS are its periodicity (it is conducted annually), its large and carefully constructed sample (about 120,000 respondents), and its well-tested questionnaire items.

Like most health care surveys, the NHIS suffers from its reliance on respondents' recall of when and how most services were used and the imprecision of self-reports of health status when compared with health examination data or medical record abstracts. The NHIS has questionnaire items on physician utilization—one with a two-week recall and one with a 12-month recall. This represents a tradeoff between response error and the stability of the estimate.

Despite its large sample size, the ability of the NHIS to disaggregate population subgroups of interest (e.g., certain minorities, the chronically ill) and other areas of concern is limited. For example, key groups with access problems, such as the homeless and migrant farm workers, are not well captured. Despite its periodicity, some key questionnaire items are not routinely included—for example, items on health insurance coverage and those that appear in various topical supplements (e.g., cancer screening, dental services) to the main survey. Despite its thoughtful design, specific questions relevant to access monitoring have not been worded to elicit the most in-depth information about access barriers, in contrast to a survey that has been specifically formulated to probe access issues. Recognizing that these limitations are not all resolvable, the committee presents recommendations in the detailed discussions (Chapter 3) of the indicators about modest changes that could maximize the utility of the survey.

In some cases the committee undertook original analyses of the NHIS.[1] Following the convention of the National Center for Health Statistics, however, estimates of persons or events are not reported in the tables in this report if the relative standard error is greater than 30 percent. Differences between estimates are discussed only in cases in which a difference was significant at at least the 5 percent level. The report also notes findings from other national surveys—specifically, the National Medical Care Expenditure Survey, the Medicare Beneficiary Survey, the National Maternal and Infant Health Survey, the Robert Wood Johnson Foundation access surveys, and the behavioral risk factor surveys of the Centers for Disease Control. These and other instruments are extremely helpful in delineating the underlying relationships that are the root causes of access barriers. They complement the routinely available NHIS data, which are the mainstay of access monitoring.

In particular, the 1987 National Medical Expenditure Survey (NMES), undertaken by the Agency for Health Care Policy and Research, explores a variety of issues that are not amenable to study under NHIS's format. Because the design involves NMES multiple interviews with the same respondent over the course of a year, an individual's changing insurance status and expenses can be tracked. The survey also provides detailed information about a person's insurance policy and physician records, which permits assessment of, for example, the effects of underinsurance on utilization.

---

[1] The Committee wishes to express its gratitude to the National Center for Health Statistics for its assistance in providing special data requests from the National Health Interview Survey.

Hospital Discharge Data

Computerized abstracts of patient discharge records organized into state data bases are increasingly available to health services researchers interested in measuring a wide range of hospital quality and cost phenomena. The committee has capitalized on recent innovations in using such data; it employed them for the comparatively new purpose of monitoring the effect access barriers can have on increasing admission rates for those who appear to be lacking the ambulatory care that might prevent hospitalization for certain conditions. The technique can also be used to detect inequities in the distribution of high-cost discretionary procedures.

This promising analytic strategy for monitoring access requires additional research and development. The lack of income data on a discharge abstract poses a methodological obstacle that is addressed by using patient zip code information. To avoid what methodologists call the "ecological fallacy," it is necessary to limit the unit of analysis to neighborhoods (characterized according to income levels) rather than patients. This means, however, that the technique cannot adequately capture access problems in localities in which the poor are dispersed throughout the population. In contrast to income information, insurance status is included on the discharge abstract under "expected source of payment." Unfortunately, this information is difficult to interpret because of the lack of good population-based data on insurance coverage. These data are needed as the basis for tracking whether admission rates per capita are related to the expected payment source. Beyond these specific problems, future studies must focus on a better understanding of the underlying reasons for delayed or inadequate care together with further scrutiny of the admission diagnoses used in the analysis.

Tumor Registries

Because early case finding through medical screening tests is a critical factor in whether people with certain types of cancer will survive, one dimension of access can be measured by the prevalence of cancers found at a late stage. The major source of this information is the tumor registry. These state/local registries record information about the pathology of tumors and other useful data such as a patient's race, age, sex, and geographic location. Like hospital discharge data bases, however, tumor registries are not established in all states and localities—which limits the ability to generalize from them to the nation as a whole. Tumor registries also lack good data on income and insurance.

Reportable Diseases

Some of the access indicators in this report rely on the tracking of certain communicable diseases. Physicians are expected to report occurrences of these diseases to their local health departments. These agencies in turn are charged with reporting them to the CDC, which routinely publishes the data. Major problems with the system are underreporting and misreporting, which occur for several reasons. Physicians' lack of understanding of the importance of sustained attention to reporting is sometimes cited as the broad reason for underreporting. Also contributing to the problem, however, are physician concerns about patient privacy, changing definitions and reporting guidelines, and the difficulties of recognizing diseases with relatively low incidences.

Claims Data

Information reported to third-party payers for the purpose of paying claims could potentially be a source of information for access monitoring. Health insurance claims contain data about utilization, health status, and costs, but they also have several major drawbacks to their use in monitoring. The major problem is an obvious one: claims data bases do not contain information about the uninsured. In addition, they are not uniform and are thus expensive to analyze. There are numerous ongoing efforts to make claims data more usable, efforts that will be considerably furthered by the movement toward widespread use of computerized medical records. In the meantime, the Health Care Financing Administration could investigate the potential contribution of the Medicaid and Medicare data bases to access monitoring. A few studies reported in the discussion of the indicators rely on analyses of these data.

CROSSCUTTING ISSUES

Most of the data bases described above are subject to two prominent concerns about obtaining information for monitoring access. One is methodological—how to obtain valid information about racial and ethnic subgroups—and the other procedural—the timely public release of data.

Race/Ethnicity

The access problems of racial and ethnic minorities have been a consistent focus of concern among health care policymakers. Inconsistent classification or misclassification of these population subgroups has frustrated both health service researchers and spokespersons for the subgroups themselves for decades. Recent results from the Hispanic Health and Nutrition Examination Survey highlight the analytic problems of lumping together Americans of Cuban, Puerto Rican, and Mexican origin who have quite different health care experiences and circumstances. Similar problems exist when Asian population subgroups are aggregated. Samples need to be of sufficient size to disentangle the effects of poverty from cultural or other characteristics specific to a group that may constitute access barriers. Oversampling in existing surveys or conducting special studies is one answer, albeit one that raises methodological and logistical issues.

Timeliness

An important rationale for access monitoring is that it allows periodic updating of indicators to identify policy and environmental changes influencing access. For this reason, making information available in a timely fashion is important, but doing so involves tradeoffs among cost, accuracy, and the response time of the indicators to changing conditions.

Data sources frequently have multiple purposes and are controlled by a variety of organizations. Therefore, the considerations involved in how the tradeoffs should be made are complex. Nevertheless, the committee's concern about lag time is real. To this end, one of the committee's recommendations addresses the need for a federal locus of authority for oversight of the monitoring process. Among other functions, such an organization would make more visible the need for and utility of data and thereby act as an advocate for the availability of timely information.

Poor race/ethnicity data and lack of timeliness are major weaknesses common to many data bases and threaten the validity inherent in the monitoring process. How the data are manipulated also demands attention. Some examples of the need for more research and analysis to further the evolution of measuring access can be cited from the committee's work. Future capacity to monitor access would be improved by creating better surrogate measures of such concepts as socioeconomic and insurance status. Further research is required to operationalize concepts like chronic disease follow-up care and excess mortality. Indices that combine data in useful ways, as in measurement of the use of prenatal care, must also be improved. The general aim over the long term should be to move toward acceptance and standardization of approaches to monitoring access to health care services.

REFERENCES

DeNeufville, J. N. 1975. *Social Indicators and Public Policy: Interactive Processes of Design and Application.* New York: Elsevier.

National Center for Health Statistics. 1989. *Current Estimates from the National Health*

Interview Survey. Series 10, No. 176. Hyattsville, Md.: National Center for Health Statistics.

Rogers, D. E. 1985. *Examining the Adequacy of a Community's Health Care.* Annual Report. Princeton, N.J.: The Robert Wood Johnson Foundation.

U.S. Department of Health and Human Services. 1991. *Healthy People 2000: National Health Promotion and Disease Prevention Objectives.* Washington, D.C.: U.S. Government Printing Office.

World Health Organization. 1981. *Development of Indicators for Monitoring Progress Towards Health for All by the Year 2000.* Geneva: WHO.

2

A Model for Monitoring Access

For most people, the frightening prospect of being unemployed, losing health insurance coverage, having inadequate insurance benefits, or living in a rural community without a physician raises one vital access-related question: Will I be able to get the care I need if I become seriously ill? At any given time in the United States, comparatively few people are seriously ill. National surveys reveal that 90 percent of Americans believe that they are in good to excellent health. Despite this record of good health, more than 75 percent of Americans have some contact with a doctor each year; only 4 percent have not seen a doctor within the past five years (National Center for Health Statistics, 1989). The reason for this seeming contradiction, of course, is that we expect more from medical care than the treatment of serious illness; we want it to keep us healthy and to ease our discomfort and disability during short bouts of illness. The care we might receive goes well beyond the physician's office to other settings and practitioners—from therapists to visiting nurses, from hospital emergency departments to public health clinics. The one-on-one interaction of provider and patient in an array of settings is often called the personal health care system.

Certain barriers can make gaining access to the personal health care system difficult. Lack of transportation, inadequate health insurance, and language difficulties are a few of the many hurdles that may stand between someone who is sick and needs health care. More broadly, barriers can create inequitable circumstances for the poor and certain minority populations. The poor and minorities not only have more difficulty getting services, but they also are in general less healthy. This may be due to not only the amount of care they receive but also the content, quality, and continuity of what care they do receive.

Access to services is not an end in and of itself. The purpose of gaining access to the personal health care system is to achieve one or more of an array of possible health outcomes—not only avoidance of untimely death and relief of acute symptoms but also maintenance of long-term functioning and relief from anxiety about the meaning of symptoms. This said, however, it should be emphasized that the relationship between desired benefits of positive health outcomes and health care services is not clear-cut. Even countries that have reduced many of the barriers faced by those in the United States by establishing universal health care still experience differences in access to health care according to social class (Illsley and Svensson, 1990). Moreover, other mechanisms in addition to medical care, such as environmental control, education, and occupational safety, contribute to the health of populations.

Despite the difficulties of sorting out the effects of health care services from those of other factors, society has a stake in monitoring how equitably its investment in health services is working, by being able to identify who has access problems and why. The challenge before the IOM committee was to identify a limited set of different personal health care services in which the connection between timely receipt of care and desired outcomes is relatively strong. These indicators can then be used to track changes in access over time and differences in access across groups in society.

DEFINING ACCESS

Access is a shorthand term used for a broad set of concerns that center on the degree to which individuals and groups are able to obtain needed services from the medical care system. Often because of difficulties in defining and measuring the term, people equate access with insurance coverage and having enough doctors and hospitals in the areas in which they live. But having insurance or nearby health care providers is no guarantee that people who need services will get them. Conversely, many who lack coverage or live in areas that appear to have shortages of health care facilities do, indeed, receive services.

Perhaps the most extensive effort to sort out the meanings of access and the related concept of equity was mounted by the 1983 President's Commission for the Study of Ethical Problems in Medicine and Biomedicine and Behavioral Science Research. The commission described society's ethical obligation to ensure access as follows: "Equitable access to health care requires that all citizens be able to secure an adequate level of care without excessive burdens" (President's Commission for the Study of Ethical Problems in Medicine and Biomedicine and Behavioral Science Research, 1983, p. 4). As the commission pointed out, however, transforming this moral obligation into reality is difficult because it involves deciding what constitutes an adequate level of care, what should be considered an excessive burden, and how to know when these standards have been reached or even exceeded.

As the IOM committee considered ways to resolve these conceptual problems, it became clear that health outcomes are as integral to the concept of access as is the use of services. Certain questions assumed central importance—for example, who is not receiving preventive services or medical treatment that would make a difference for health status? Who is not receiving care that eases pain, improves functioning, or alleviates anxiety? With equity of access to health services, the answers to these questions should not be affected by race, ethnic origin, income, geographical location, or insurance status.

Based on these considerations, the committee defined access as follows: **the timely use of personal health services to achieve the best possible health outcomes.** Importantly, this definition relies on both the use of health services and on health outcomes to provide yardsticks for judging whether access has been achieved. The test of equity of access involves determining whether there are systematic differences in use and outcome among groups in society and whether these differences are the result of financial or other barriers to care.

A standard of "the best possible health outcome" is admittedly an ideal goal. Particularly in a society that limits the resources devoted to health care, all that medical science can offer is an optimistic target, unattainable for every patient. Social critics commenting on the health care scene have reminded us from time to time that, even if we could afford it, more medical services are not necessarily a good thing, nor are more services frequently the best road to good health for a society faced with tradeoffs about the best social investments it could make (Evans and Stoddart, 1990; Illich, 1975).

In applying its definition of access the committee sought to occupy a practical middle ground between all care that people might want or believe they needed and the view that medical care can make an important difference in people's lives. The definition forces us to identify those areas of medical care in which services influence health status and then to ask whether the relatively poorer outcomes of some population groups can be explained by problems related to access. The definition also emphasizes the need to move beyond standard approaches that rely mainly on enumerating the presence of health care providers, the number of uninsured, or encounters with health care providers to detect access problems.

For a health outcome to be a useful indicator of access problems, one must be able to take into account many factors other than medical care that may contribute to differences in outcome among groups, including those factors that may not be easily overcome by medical care. This problem can be addressed by focusing on health outcomes for which the connection between services and desired benefits is as unambiguous as possible. For example, it is known that Pap smears allow early diagnosis of cervical cancer, which leads to better chances of survival. Thus, the incidence of invasive cervical cancer, an outcome measure, may be a good indicator of access to primary care services. In contrast, mortality from pancreatic cancer would not make a good access indicator because there is no reliable screening test for the disease nor is there a good prognosis for survival even with early detection.

Employing the utilization of health care services as an indicator of health care access also has limitations. Some people are prone to overuse medical care, whereas others may underuse it for reasons that have little to do with access barriers. Others use more services because they need more. For example, the poor may use a greater amount of care because they are more likely to have health problems than those with higher income levels. To interpret utilization indicators unambiguously, efforts must be made to account for need and appropriateness of services.

MEASURING ACCESS

Indicators

To the extent that they reflect objective conditions and social values, indicators can mobilize sociopolitical pressures to raise the overall health levels of the population. They can also provide insight into how well medical knowledge is being applied in a given society to a given population. They offer as well a way of tracking how well a society is discharging its responsibilities for the organization and delivery of health care (Elinson, 1974).

The systematic and periodic reporting of statistics to describe social change and inform policy choices is not new, although it came into its own as the "social indicator movement" in the 1960s (DeNeufville, 1975; Land and Spilerman, 1972). Although some might argue that the widespread enthusiasm of the 1960s for social indicators has waned, the notion of indicators to measure progress in the health arena has continued to be strong, as demonstrated by the U.S. Year 2000 health objectives and the World Health Organization Year 2000 activities (U.S. Public Health Service, 1991).

Generally, an indicator is a sign or symptom that points to the existence of a phenomenon or to a change of status in a phenomenon over time (Andrews, 1989). The phenomenon of interest in the IOM Access Monitor-

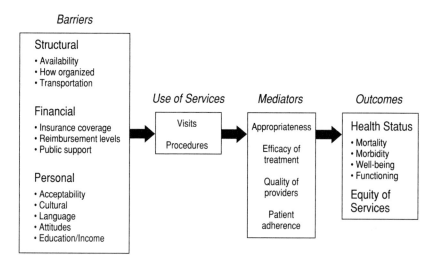

FIGURE 2-1   Model of access to personal health care services.

ing Project, depicted graphically in Figure 2-1, is the dynamic of participation in the personal health care system: namely, that access problems are created when barriers cause underuse of services, which in turn leads to poor outcomes. In particular, the committee was interested in identifying, quantifying, and relating aspects of three parts of the model—barriers, utilization, and outcomes—that point to problems that individuals or groups have in gaining access to the health care system. The challenge for the committee was to find indicators of utilization and outcomes that vary according to the financial, structural, and personal barriers discussed below.

Indicators have been likened to an automobile temperature gauge. "Even though it reports only one thing—coolant temperature at a specific place in the engine—and does not give temperature readings at all points in the engine, it nevertheless does serve as a useful indicator of the general state of the engine with respect to temperature" (Andrews, 1989, p. 27). Similarly, the access monitoring indicators recommended by the committee are intended to sense when and where access problems occur in the personal health care system. They cannot explain the exact causes of these problems, but they do provide a basis for generating theories about why differences in access exist among populations. Indicators "are indirect or partial measures of a complex situation, but if measured sequentially over time they can indicate direction and speed of change and serve to compare different areas or groups of people at the same moment in time" (World Health Organization, 1981, p. 12).

Indicators will not always move in the same direction. Some may increase, some may decline, and others may show no change. Although this makes overall assessments more complicated, it can be useful for highlighting problems and gains in specific areas.

It is important not to confuse the purposes that drive the development and use of indicators with those of research studies that seek to explicate the causes of access differentials among population subgroups. A major reason to disaggregate access indicators is to be able to track subgroups of policy interest, such as racial and ethnic groups, the uninsured, and the poor. Researchers, however, are engaged in seeking to identify all the possible variables of interest and to determine their relative contribution to the variability seen in access measures. That information ultimately is quite useful for developing and interpreting indicators.

The literature on social indicators makes a distinction between descriptive and analytic indicators, the latter being grounded in theoretical models in which an interrelationship among variables is explicit. For example, the interrelated components of economic models are indicators whose variation tells us a great deal about the functioning of the economic system (Rossi, 1980). In the case of health care access models, the committee has provided a framework for the access indicators, but it will require years of tracking and further research to begin to approach the sophistication of economic models.

Utilization Indicators

One of the most common ways of determining whether access to health care has been realized is to look at the frequency of visits to a health care provider or the use of medical procedures. Surveys attempting to explore the nature of access have investigated various properties of utilization: who provided the care (physician, dentist); the care setting (office, outpatient department); the purpose of the visit (preventive, curative, custodial); and, finally, the frequency and continuity of use (Aday et al., 1980).

The IOM Access Monitoring Project sought to capture these dimensions of utilization in the selection of indicators. The utilization indicators encompass the services of various types of providers in different settings, including primary and specialty physicians and dentists. Data permitting, it is the committee's aim to broaden the utilization measures to other types of providers. Indirectly, these services are captured by outcome measures that should reflect effective services of nonphysician practitioners. For example, effective prenatal care services for poor pregnant teenagers should incorporate nutrition services, which may be provided by dieticians. In addition to type of provider and setting, the committee chose indicators that would cut across the personal health care system to include, at a minimum, prevention, early case finding, chronic disease care, surgical procedures, and primary care visits.

Outcome Indicators

For all their usefulness, utilization rates, if used alone to gauge equity of access, can be problematic. A poor mother who brings her asthmatic child to a clinic but cannot afford to purchase the prescribed medication may have a visit recorded, but few would consider that she had adequate access. A poor pregnant woman with a drug addiction requires many more services than most middle-class women if she is to deliver a healthy baby. A physician may be reluctant to order an expensive diagnostic test for an uninsured patient while erring on the side of overutilization for someone with adequate insurance. Thus, the poor and uninsured may enter the medical system, but it is difficult to tell whether they receive the services they need. An additional limitation of using utilization of health care services as a way to measure access is that it is frequently impossible to track all the services people need when they need them, especially for complex chronic diseases.

Looking at health care outcomes is a complementary approach to measuring access. Outcomes can be measured in terms of survival; states of physiological, physical, and emotional health; and satisfaction (Lohr, 1988). Carefully selected outcome indicators, based on such measures as death rates, disease incidence, and conditions that require hospitalization, indirectly provide clues about access barriers that may be impeding appropriate care.

Health researchers and policymakers interested in assuring and improving quality of care have focused their attention on outcome measures as a way of assessing it. For example, a list of diseases amenable to treatment were identified in the 1970s as "sentinel" measures of quality (Rutstein et al., 1976). They were sentinel in the sense that high rates of death from these diseases indicated a quality-of-care problem. This idea was adapted to identify conditions that were sentinel for access problems—a technique described in Chapter 3.

Utilization and Its Relationship to Health Care

Mediating Factors

Access is only one of several mediating factors that stand between the use of health care services and desired health outcomes. These mediating factors must be taken into account in selecting indicators and in drawing conclusions about equity of access. In any particular case a given service may not have a positive outcome because (1) it is inappropriate for that patient, (2) some percentage of all disease processes may not respond to the appropriate treatment, (3) the treatment is of questionable efficacy, (4) the disease defeats the best that medical care can offer, (5) the diagnostic and treatment skills of the provider are below acceptable standards, or (6) the patient does not follow the treatment regimen.

The effects of the first three factors can be minimized by selecting services and related outcomes for which the value of a service is relatively unquestioned because, on average, the intervention has demonstrated benefits. In addition, there should be little variation in practice styles that affect when and how to intervene medically.

The second two mediating factors are more difficult to deal with. It is known that in some instances the poor receive care from so-called Medicaid mills, which provide perfunctory services of questionable quality. Even when the poor receive services from hospital outpatient departments or emergency rooms, or in public health clinics, the care may be fragmentary and lack continuity from one visit to the next. These examples may more properly fall under the heading of quality than access, but often the two concepts overlap.

Lack of patient adherence to treatment regimens can range from refusal to take a prescribed medicine to the drug addict's inability to make major lifestyle changes. The distinction between the personal responsibility of the patient for his or her own health and the sociocultural barriers that interfere with good health service outcomes is often difficult to make. How far should the health care system go to compensate for personal factors that may inhibit a patient from complying with the provider's advice? Most would agree that a clinic in the midst of a Southeast Asian refugee community should find a way to have translators available and that the clinic staff should be knowledgeable about the patients' cultural attitudes. In other situations the responsibilities of those who provide health care are less clear. The committee hopes to stimulate productive debate on the factors that mediate the effects of health care services as people attempt to interpret the results of access monitoring.

In summary, no matter how generally efficacious a particular health service may be, a good health care outcome cannot always be guaranteed. The most important consideration is whether people have the opportunity for a good outcome—especially in those instances in which medical care can make a difference. When those opportunities are systematically denied to groups in society because they face barriers to care, there is an access problem that needs to be addressed.

Barriers to Access

There are three primary types of barriers to health care. *Structural barriers* are impediments to medical care directly related to the number, type, concentration, location, or organizational configuration of health care providers. *Financial barriers* may restrict access either by inhibiting the ability of patients to pay for needed medical services or by discouraging physicians and hospitals from treating patients of limited means. *Personal and cultural barriers* may inhibit people who need medical attention from seeking it or, once they obtain care, from following recommended posttreatment guidelines.

These barriers interact in complicated ways. The simple presence or absence of a barrier does not guarantee that one can predict whether services can be obtained. For example, many women without insurance receive prenatal services from community health centers or public health clinics. In some cases these services may better meet their needs than the care women with insurance coverage receive. In addition, many who live in areas designated as having a shortage of health care professionals actually have physicians available to them locally or are willing to travel to the nearest physician. In contrast, many people live in areas with high physician-to-population ratios but are unable to secure needed services (Berk et al., 1984).

Structural Barriers

The post-World War II solution to health care access problems was to expand the basic supply of hospital beds and later, in the 1960s, the supply of health care professionals. The federal government adopted a policy of capacity building at the local level partly in recognition of the fact that the recently enacted Medicare and Medicaid entitlements would strain the health care delivery system by increasing the demand for medical care. Community health centers, the national health service corps, and other programs designed to increase the number of health care professionals in underserved areas were seen as mechanisms by which local communities could take advantage of the broader availability of public insurance. The legacy of this period was to measure access in terms of beds, facilities, and providers in relation to population.

With the strain that growing demand placed on public budgets, however, the 1960s gave way to a move from expansion to constraining capacity in the 1970s through regulatory mechanisms such as certificate-of-need programs. During the 1980s, disillusionment with planning and regulatory approaches led to greater reliance on market forces to control costs.

How health care resources are organized in the 1990s may be as important for improving access as the production of hospital beds and health professions schools was in an earlier period. Much of the substance of the current national discourse on organizing care derives from the objective that people neither over- nor underutilize care but instead receive care that is appropriate to their condition. The aim is to improve access by redistributing health resources in society—not so as to deny the haves for the sake of the have-nots—but to improve quality for all with judicious use of health care. For the insured with severe or multiple chronic diseases, access to the complicated mix of services that will keep them functioning optimally may necessitate some type of case manager or coordinator. For the poor and uninsured, case management takes on the added meaning of being able to meld public health and social services with personal health care (Enthoven, 1988). Hopes are being pinned to the notion that devising the best mix of risk sharing among payers, patients, and providers will result in a good balance between cost control and quality.

The implicit lesson from this brief historical overview is that most structural barriers to access have their roots in the way health care is financed. Despite a greatly enlarged physician force and the existence of some 600 community health centers, many of today's poor still find it difficult to identify physicians who will accept Medicaid. A major reason for this dilemma is Medicaid's low reimbursement rates. Practitioners seek locations in which they can generate sufficient revenues to support a practice, and these areas often are not easily reached by those living in rural areas or urban neighborhoods with a high concentration of poverty. Racial discrimination and the disinclination of providers to offer discounts and charity care may be other explanations.

Patients who do not succeed in identifying a private physician or health center most often rely on local emergency rooms and hospital outpatient clinics for their primary medical care. Some hospitals have tailored the organization of their services to accommodate this patient population. By its nature, however, emergency care lacks the necessary continuity to deal with many medical problems that are treated more adequately when there is a regular provider of care.

Financial Barriers

The costs of health care, which have risen faster than most services in the economy and faster than real incomes, have made it virtually infeasible for most people to pay directly for any sizable portion of their medical bills when illness strikes. Even maternity care—once an affordable service on a middle-class income—is almost an unthinkable expense now without health insurance. Added to this is the fact that there are growing numbers of families in poverty. The 13.5 percent poverty rate in 1990—up from 12.8 percent a year earlier—is higher than at any time in the 1970s. The most recent high, however, was the 15 percent rate in 1983 (Bureau of the Census, 1991).

The ability to pay for medical care is closely linked to having public or private health care coverage. Financial barriers to health care access may manifest themselves in several ways: eligibility/insurability, benefit coverage, and reimbursement levels. When insurance fails, it is the responsibility of direct service delivery programs to act as a safety net.

The three major surveys that have regularly monitored the size of the uninsured population all have shown an upward trend of about 25 percent over the past 10 or more years even though they differ somewhat on the exact counts. The National Medical Expenditure Survey in 1977 recorded that 12.3 percent of the population under 65 years of age was uninsured, a proportion that increased to 15.5 percent a decade later (Short et al., 1988). The National Health Interview Survey also reported an increase—from 12.5 percent in 1980 to 15.7 percent in 1989. The Current Population Survey (CPS) of the Census Bureau showed increases throughout the 1980s, although a change in the wording of the questionnaire in 1986 makes trend interpretation difficult. Recently, the CPS reported that the proportion of nonelderly uninsured was 16.6 percent of the population. This 1990 figure was an increase from the 1988 level of 15.9 percent with no insurance (Employee Benefits Research Institute, 1992).

The poor and minorities bear a heavy share of the burden of lack of insurance. In 1990, 55 percent of the uninsured were in families with annual incomes of less than $20,000. Although blacks constitute only 12.7 percent of the U.S. population, they represent 17.4 percent of those without health care coverage. The corresponding figures for Hispanics are 9.3 percent and 19.6 percent (Employee Benefits Research Institute, 1992).

The issue of health care coverage is a question not only of the absence or presence of insurance but also of underinsurance—the depth or adequacy of coverage. As the cost of medical care relative to income soars, individuals find it increasingly difficult to maintain the breadth of their coverage. Furthermore, employers are likely to shift some proportion of premium cost increases to their employees through the employee contribution route and benefit restrictions. Underinsurance could affect access when policies do not cover preexisting medical conditions, when they require copayments and deductibles that cause delays in necessary care, or when they fail to cover certain categories of benefits (e.g., mental health services). Underinsurance is a difficult concept to gauge operationally because there is an inherent value judgment involved in setting criteria for what services should be covered and how much in out-of-pocket costs should be borne by individuals. In many cases cost sharing has been promoted as a way to reduce overutilization. In terms of access, underinsurance is interpretable only in

TABLE 2-1   Percentage of the Elderly Covered Only by Medicare by Race, Selected Years

Race	1980	1984	1989
Total	22.7	20.0	16.8
Race[a]			
White	21.0	18.5	14.7
Black	40.6	34.5	37.9
Ratio black/white	1.9	1.9	2.6

[a]Includes persons not covered by private insurance or Medicaid.

SOURCES: Unpublished data from the National Center for Health Statistics; National Health Interview Surveys, National Center for Health Statistics (1990c).

the context of the economic circumstances of an individual in relation to the extent of coverage in his or her specific insurance policy.

Because most elderly people are entitled to Medicare benefits, they are frequently neglected in discussions of access. But Medicare benefits are not comprehensive; consequently, most elderly also carry supplemental private insurance. As Table 2-1 illustrates, less than 20 percent of the elderly have only Medicare. The table also shows that there are some important differences by race, suggesting the potential for underinsurance of these groups and the consequent need to monitor their access problems. In addition to these long-standing issues of comprehensiveness, the effect of recent reforms, including physician reimbursement rules, on access is something that the Physician Payment Review Commission set up by Congress is planning to monitor.

The millions of Americans without health insurance coverage do not necessarily go without care. Much of their care is financed through direct service delivery programs supported by federal, state, and local budgets or is delivered by institutional and individual providers in the form of free or reduced-price services. Included are the budgets of public hospitals, health department clinics, facilities run by the Department of Veterans Affairs, and community health center clinics. A host of special programs enacted by states and localities operate as a health safety net for those who do not qualify for Medicaid. This safety net can be threatened by government budget cuts or the inability of programs to keep pace with increased demand when there are downturns in the economy.

Personal and Cultural Barriers

When population subgroups that share personal characteristics—such as education levels or attitudes—systematically underuse services that make a difference to health, there is good reason to believe that a problem exists in equity of access. The problem can often be addressed by modifying structural or financial barriers in ways that compensate for patient lack of education or negative patient attitudes about the way care is organized.

The importance of considering the effect of personal and cultural factors on access is heightened by the nation's changing demography. For example, in the late 1980s the foreign-born portion of the U.S. population reached 7 percent from a low of 4.9 percent in 1970. The number of immigrants living in the United States is at an all-time high of 18 million (Fix and Passel, 1991).

Other industrialized nations that have addressed many of the fundamental financial and structural barriers to access are now focusing on cultural determinants of service use and health outcomes that contribute to inequalities in their societies. As Lagasse and his colleagues (1990) note,

> Like motherhood and childbirth, and their related practices, disease has to be considered in a cultural context. . . . We define "health culture" as a set of rules—either implicit or explicit—which determine the behavior of social subjects in relation to their health. Those rules may be obligations or interdictions, repulsions or desires, likes or dislikes. They may be determinants for the body's use or the body's perceptual status, the distribution of the roles inside the family concerning health and disease, the choice of alternative ways to solve health problems (traditional or scientific approach, official or "parallel" medicines), the definition of the limits between normal and abnormal situations in the somatic, psychological, psychosocial, familial or other domains. (p. 238)

For various subpopulations in the United States, insurance and provider availability are necessary but not sufficient for obtaining access to health care. Migrant farm workers, refugees, newly arrived immigrants, the functionally illiterate, and the homeless—who are likely to have worse-than-average health status—may need translators, outreach workers, and sensitive practitioners to overcome cultural and other barriers to care that could make a difference in their health status.

Much recent research on access problems in the Hispanic and black communities has sought to disentangle the role of cultural factors from other barriers. Most of these studies have found that financial and structural barriers, rather than lack of acculturation, explain most differences in the use of health care services. It has been argued that access problems faced by non-English-speaking patients are more appropriately viewed as a structural defect in the health care delivery system rather than as part of some larger cultural construct.

The Relationship of Access Barriers to Indicators

As is evident from the foregoing discussion, there are no clear demarcation lines among the types of barriers to access. They are highly interrelated—part of the complex processes involved in seeking health care and achieving good outcomes from that care. Nevertheless, they allow us to begin thinking about how measures of access (utilization and outcome) vary according to measures of equity (financing, structural, and personal/cultural factors). The number of uninsured, poor, and ethnic and racial minorities is growing. How well has the health care system adjusted to these changing realities?

In the next chapter the committee proposes a set of outcome and utilization indicators. The extent and direction of change in these indicators should reflect the efforts of policymakers to reduce barriers to care.

REFERENCES

Aday, L. A., Anderson, R., and Fleming, G. 1980. *Health Care in the U.S.: Equitable for Whom?* Beverly Hills, Calif.: Sage Publications.

Andrews, F. 1989. Developing indicators of health promotion: Contribution from the social indicators movement. In: *Health Promotion Indicators and Actions.* S. B. Kar, ed. New York: Springer Publishing Co., pp. 29-49.

Berk, M. L., Bernstein, A., and Taylor, A. K. 1984. The use and availability of medical care in health manpower shortage areas. *Inquiry* 20(Winter):369-380.

Bureau of the Census, U.S. Department of Commerce. 1991. *Statistical Abstract of the United States, 1991*, 11th ed. Washington, D.C.: U.S. Government Printing Office, pp. 462-466.

DeNeufville, J. I. 1975. *Social Indicators and Public Policy: Interactive Processes of Design and Application.* Amsterdam: Elsevier.

Elinson, J. 1974. Toward sociomedical health indicators. *Social Indicators Research* 1:59-71.

Employee Benefits Research Institute. 1992. *Sources of Health Insurance and Characteristics of the Uninsured: Analysis of the March 1991 Current Population Study.* An EBRI Special Report and Issue. Brief No. 123. Washington, D.C.: EBRI.

Enthoven, A. C. 1988. Managed competition: An agenda for action. *Health Affairs* 7(3):25-47.

Evans, R. G., and Stoddart, G. L. 1990. Producing health, consuming health care. *Social Science and Medicine* 31:1347-1364.

Fix, M., and Passel, J. 1991. *The Door Remains Open. Recent Immigration to the United States and a Preliminary Analysis of the Immigration Act of 1990.* Document No. PRIP-VI-14. Washington, D.C.: The Urban Institute.

Illich, I. 1975. *Medical Nemesis: The Expropriation of Health.* Toronto: Mclleland and Stewart.

Illsley, R. and Svensson, P. G., eds. 1990. Health Inequities in Europe. Special issue of *Social Science and Medicine* 31:229-236.

Lagasse, R., Humblet, P. C., Lenaerts, A., Godin, I., and Moens, G. F. 1990. Health and social inequities in Belgium. *Social Science and Medicine* 31:237-248.

Land, K. C. and Spilerman, S., eds. 1972. *Social Indicator Models.* New York: Russell Sage Foundation.

Lohr, K. N. 1988. Outcome measurement concepts and questions. *Inquiry* 25:37-50.

National Center for Health Statistics. 1989. *Current Estimates from the National Health Interview Survey.* Series 10, No. 176. Hyattsville, Md.: NCHS.

President's Commission for the Study of Ethical Problems in Medicine and Biomedicine and Behavioral Science Research. 1983. *Securing Access to Health Care: The Ethical Implications of Differences in the Availability of Health Services*, vol. 1. Washington, D.C.: President's Commission.

Rossi, R. J. 1980. *The Handbook of Social Indicators: Sources, Characteristics, and Analysis.* New York: Garland STPM Press.

Rutstein, D. D., Berenberg, W. B., Chalmers, T. C., et al. 1976. Measuring the quality of medical care: A clinical method. *New England Journal of Medicine* 294:582-588.

Short, P. F., Monheit, A. C., and Beauregard, K. 1988. *Uninsured Americans: A 1987 Profile.* Rockville, Md.: National Center for Health Services Research and Health Care Technology Assessment.

U.S. Public Health Service. 1991. *Healthy People: National Health Promotion and Disease Prevention Objectives.* DHHS Pub. No. (PHS) 91-50212. Washington, D.C.: U.S. Government Printing Office.

World Health Organization. 1981. *Development of Indicators for Monitoring Progress Towards Health for All by the Year 2000.* Geneva: WHO.

3

Using Indicators to Monitor National Objectives for Health Care

As noted earlier, the committee believes that assessing access to health care requires more than a simple tally of the use of services. The content and appropriateness of those services also must be estimated. Implicit in the committee's definition of access is the idea that certain services improve health. Thus, for many, if not most, personal health care services, there is an expectation of benefit, and that benefit extends beyond such obviously important outcomes as avoiding death to more subtle quality-of-life values like physical and social functioning.

With these concepts in mind, the committee focused on access problems that it believes, if corrected, are most likely to lead to improved health outcomes on a wide scale. Indicators were then identified that could be used to measure changes in the degree of access to specific health care services. After considerable discussion, the committee agreed on a list of 15 indicators, which were grouped into several distinct categories. The categories define a set of national objectives for the personal health care system, with each set of indicators providing a means of assessing progress toward a specific objective. The objectives are as follows: (1) promoting successful birth outcomes; (2) reducing the incidence of vaccine-preventable childhood diseases; (3) early detection and diagnosis of treatable diseases; (4) reducing the effects of chronic diseases and prolonging life; and (5) reducing morbidity and pain through providing timely and appropriate treatment. Table 3-1 shows for each objective the related indicators, how they are measured, and the latest year for which data are available.

TABLE 3-1 Access Indicators

Objective/ Indicator	Measure	Latest Data Available
1. Promoting successful birth outcomes		
Adequacy of prenatal care (u)	Percentage of pregnant women obtaining adequate care	1988
Infant mortality (o)	Children who die before first birthday (per 1,000 live births)	1990
Low birthweight (o)	Percentage of infants born weighing less than 2,500 grams	1988
Congenital syphilis (o)	Cases per 100,000 population	1990
2. Reducing the incidence of vaccine- preventable childhood diseases		
Immunization rates (u)	Percentage of preschool children vaccinated	1985
Incidence of preventable childhood communicable diseases (diphtheria, measles, mumps, pertussis, polio, rubella, and tetanus) (o)	Cases per 100,000 population	1989
3. Early detection and diagnosis of treatable diseases		
Breast and cervical cancer screening (u)	Percentage of women undergoing procedure in given period	
	• Clinical breast exam	1987
	• Mammogram	1990
	• Pap test	1987
Incidence of late-stage breast and cervical cancers (o)	Percentage of tumors diagnosed at late stages	
	• Breast cancer	1983–1987
	• Cervical cancer	1983–1987

continued on next page

TABLE 3-1 *Continued*

Objective/ Indicator	Measure	Latest Data Available
4. Reducing the effects of chronic diseases and prolonging life		
Chronic disease follow-up care (u)	Average number of physician contacts annually by those in fair to poor health; proportion with no physician contacts in previous year	1989
Use of high-cost discretionary care (u)	Admissions for referral-sensitive surgeries	1988
Avoidable hospitalization for chronic diseases (o)	Admissions for ambulatory-care-sensitive chronic conditions	1988
Access-related excess mortality (o)	Number of deaths per 100,000 population estimated to be due to access problems	1988
5. Reducing morbidity and pain through timely and appropriate treatment		
Acute medical care (u)	Percentage of individuals with acute illness who have no physician contact	1989
Dental services (u)	Average number of dental visits per year	1989
Avoidable hospitalization for acute conditions (o)	Admissions for ambulatory-care-sensitive conditions	1988

u, utilization; o, outcome.

The sections that follow discuss one or more utilization and outcome indicators for each objective. An indicator is first defined and the rationale for including it in the report is presented. This is followed by a subsection on measurement and an analysis of any methodological or measurement problems. A third subsection discusses overall trends in the data related to the particular indicator and, where possible, includes specific information on racial and ethnic groups. It also describes and provides data on barriers to access faced by various groups (the uninsured, the less educated, etc.) in the population. The final subsection contains the committee's recommendations.

The committee did not attempt to develop its own quantitative goals for the indicator measures. Where possible, the Year 2000 Health Objectives for the Nation goals are cited as a benchmark and to indicate existing consensus about the desired levels of service use or health status. Time series data are explored to indicate improvement or lack of improvement over the past decade. Finally, comparisons among population subgroups are made and constitute a major focus for interpretations.

OBJECTIVE 1: PROMOTING SUCCESSFUL BIRTH OUTCOMES

Utilization Indicator: Adequacy of Prenatal Care

Prenatal care consists of medical services and procedures intended to monitor and maintain the health of mother and fetus from conception to delivery. For the purposes of this report, prenatal care at a minimum consists of periodic examinations to screen for and manage health risks to the mother and developing fetus. Prenatal visits comprise an accurate medical history, physical exam (including a check of blood pressure), and laboratory tests (including tests for serum glucose levels, sexually transmitted diseases, and cervical cancer).

The results of these periodic visits will determine the necessary degree of monitoring and intervention. For example, a woman found to have gestational diabetes, abnormal weight gain, signs of premature labor, or preeclampsia (hypertension of pregnancy) may require more frequent visits to the obstetrician or certain nonstandard medical procedures or tests. Women at high risk for poor pregnancy outcomes—such as those who smoke, those who suffer from malnutrition or nutritional imbalance, or those who are addicted to drugs or alcohol—may need to take part in a wide range of medical, health education, and social service programs. The content of prenatal care can vary widely depending on the patient's needs, what health care services are available, and which of the available services the patient chooses to take advantage of.

Extensive efforts have been made to evaluate the components of prenatal care. The Public Health Service's Expert Panel on the Content of Prenatal Care has analyzed a large constellation of services and procedures that constitute prenatal care. The panel reviewed the scientific and medical literature to determine the efficacy and appropriate timing of more than 130 individual components of prenatal care (Public Health Service Expert Panel on the Content of Prenatal Care, 1989). Another major recent effort to define the content of prenatal care is the seventh edition of *Standards for Obstetric-Gynecological Services* published in 1989 by the American College of Obstetricians and Gynecologists. Numerous studies have shown the link between the timing, amount, and content of prenatal care and successful birth outcomes. Prenatal care also has been shown to be cost effective, particularly for poorly educated, low-income women who otherwise might incur significant direct medical expenses for the care of their low-birthweight infants (Institute of Medicine, 1985, 1988; Office of Technology Assessment, 1988).

The committee realizes that a woman's general health status prior to becoming pregnant has a significant impact on the course and outcome of her pregnancy. Nevertheless, the prenatal period is of critical importance because a host of interventions are known to make a significant difference in the outcome of a pregnancy, regardless of the mother's prior health history.

Two aspects of a woman's access to health care services and her health-seeking behavior prior to pregnancy are worth noting. First is the use and content of so-called preconception medical care, which has been shown to have a direct influence on the later use of prenatal care services. Women are much more likely to use prenatal care services during their pregnancy when the pregnancy is planned (and the child is wanted) than when it is unplanned or mistimed (and the child is unwanted). Noting that more than half of all pregnancies in the United States are unwanted, the IOM Committee to Study Outreach for Prenatal Care concluded that more extensive use of family planning services (a "preconception" service) would result in reduced rates of late entry into prenatal care (Institute of Medicine, 1988).

The second aspect is the role, indirect and direct, that nutrition services, particularly the Special Supplemental Food Program for Women, Infants, and Children (WIC), play in improving maternal and infant health. WIC is among those services ancillary to prenatal care that have great potential for enhancing the outcome of pregnancy. There is considerable evidence that WIC participation reduces rates of low birthweight and infant mortality (Caan et al., 1987; Centers for Disease Control, 1978; Coit, 1977; Collins et al., 1985; Food Research Action Center, 1991; Kennedy and Kotelchuck, 1984; Rush et al., 1988b; Schramm, 1986). Other research (Kotelchuck et al., 1984; Rush et al., 1988a; U.S. Department of Agriculture, 1990) has shown that women who participate in the WIC program enter early prenatal care more often than women who are eligible but do not participate. A large proportion of women who are eligible to participate in the WIC program do not do so. In 1984, for example, although some 7.5 million women, infants, and children were eligible, only slightly more than 3 million received WIC benefits (U.S. Department of Agriculture, 1987). It is generally believed that lack of knowledge about available benefits and administrative barriers to enrollment are in great measure to blame for lack of access to the program.

Measuring the Indicator

The primary source for data on prenatal care is the birth certificate. The data are reported by states annually to the National Center for Health Statistics (NCHS). Another important source of information about prenatal care is the 1988 National Maternal and Infant Health Survey (National Center for Health Statistics, 1991), which gathered data from mothers and their health care providers.

There are two aspects of prenatal care that are frequently measured: its initiation and frequency. When a woman first obtains prenatal care is important because care initiated early in a pregnancy has the best chance of preventing or treating medical conditions that could potentially harm the mother or fetus. Similarly, how often a women receives prenatal care is important, too, because periodic monitoring (with frequency determined by need) is essential for ensuring a good pregnancy outcome.

Because many insurance plans do not cover prenatal care and because Medicaid does not reimburse for these services at levels high enough to encourage all providers to participate, income is an important barrier to access. However, securing direct evidence of the link between income and access to care on a routine basis is difficult since income information is not reported on birth certificates. The Health Resources and Services Administration is testing the feasibility of combining the information provided on birth certificates with income data by zip code from the Census Bureau to estimate the income levels of women who use varying quantities of prenatal care services. Preliminary results from a pilot study in New York City indicate that living in lower-income neighborhoods is correlated with less use of prenatal care (Zeitel et al., 1991).

Several factors may affect the accuracy and usefulness of various measures of prenatal care. For example, none of the several measurement methodologies in widespread use defines in any precise way the components of a typical prenatal care visit (Institute of Medicine, 1988). In addition, several measurement methods rely for data collection on the memories of pregnant women or on their medical records, both of which can be faulty. Even the accuracy of birth certificates, used by the NCHS to generate most of the available information about prenatal care, has been called into question (National Center for Health Statistics, 1983; see also NCHS, 1980a).

In addition to these generic problems, each of the three most common approaches to assessing the use of prenatal care has specific limitations. Studies that simply count the number of prenatal care visits tell nothing about the distribution of those visits throughout the pregnancy. Analyses that focus on when prenatal care was begun fail to reveal whether that care had any continuity. Moreover, indices of prenatal care that combine the number of visits and timing of prenatal care with other variables (in the case of the modified Kessner index, for example, with gestational age) can be confounded by incomplete or missing data for one or more variables (Alexander et al., 1991). In short, no currently available method for measuring the use of prenatal care services is without its drawbacks.

Trends in the Data

The committee decided that the most valuable overall indicator of utilization is the percentage of women receiving adequate prenatal care as measured by the modified Kessner index. Although it recognizes the problems with the Kessner index, the committee believes that by combining early initiation of care with the number of visits (adjusted for gestation), the index provides the most appropriate standard of the measures currently and widely available.

Table 3-2 displays the percent distribution of births by adequacy of care for 1986–1988 as measured by the modified Kessner index. For all races, slightly less than 70 percent of all women received adequate prenatal care in each of the three years. In each year nearly three-quarters of white women but only one-half of black women received adequate care. Comparable national data from earlier years are not available. Although the relative differences are small, improvement was greater for whites (0.9 percent) than for blacks (0.1 percent)—a trend that should be watched closely in future years. The NCHS plans to update the Kessner index annually. Beginning in 1989, all states are reporting the data necessary to construct the index.

Trend data are available to indicate the percentage of women who begin prenatal care in the first trimester, a key component of the modified Kessner Index. As Table 3-3 indicates, approximately 75 percent of all U.S. women begin prenatal care at that time. The comparable figure for white women is approximately 80 percent and for black women 60 percent. The table also shows that the percentage of women receiving early care increased steadily during the 1970s (from 67.9 percent for all races in 1970 to 75.9 percent in 1979) but remained static between 1980 and 1988. As the final column in the table indicates, the gap in the use of early prenatal services between white and black women, after decreasing rapidly during the 1970s, has worsened slightly since 1980.

Table 3-4 indicates the percentage of women, by race/ethnicity of the

TABLE 3-2 Percent Distribution of U.S. Births by Adequacy of Care (Modified Kessner Index), 1986–1988

Care Level	All Races	Black	White
Adequate			
1986	68.4	50.6	72.6
1987	68.7	50.7	73.2
1988	68.9	50.7	73.5
Intermediate			
1986	23.6	34.2	21.0
1987	23.2	33.6	20.6
1988	23.1	33.8	20.4
Inadequate			
1986	8.0	15.3	6.3
1987	8.1	15.7	6.2
1988	8.0	15.5	6.1

SOURCE: National Center for Health Statistics, based on data from 49 reporting states and the District of Columbia.

mother, seeking early prenatal care. The percentage for all races for 1988 was 75.9; however, the percentages by ethnic group varied from less than 60 percent for Native Americans and Mexican Americans and 61.1 percent for blacks to 82.4 percent for Chinese, 83.4 percent for Cubans, and 86.3 percent for Japanese. Less than 65 percent of Puerto Rican and Central and South American women living in the United States had early prenatal visits in 1988. The wide variations by race and ethnicity have been constant over the past decade (U.S. Public Health Service, 1991).

The existence of a broad range of barriers to the use of prenatal care services has been extensively documented. Indeed, several years ago IOM prepared a review of much of the relevant literature, grouping the barriers into four categories: (1) financial (including insurance or lack thereof, eligibility for insurance coverage, scope and depth of insurance coverage, and Medicaid coverage); (2) inadequate capacity of the personal health care system (including not only private physicians but also factors influencing such organized health care settings as hospital outpatient departments and community and migrant health centers); (3) organizational aspects of prenatal services (including links among various programs that furnish prenatal care); and (4) cultural and personal factors (including care-seeking behavior, views about the importance of prenatal care, and drug and alcohol abuse) (Institute of Medicine, 1988).

Measuring the organizational factors that influence the quality and con-

TABLE 3-3   Percentage of U.S. Women Receiving Early Prenatal Care,[a] by Race, 1970–1988

			Nonwhite		Ratio
Year	All Races	White	Black	Total	White/Black
1970	67.9	72.4	44.3	46.0	1.63
1971	68.6	73.0	44.3	48.1	1.65
1972	69.4	73.6	49.0	50.6	1.50
1973	70.8	74.9	51.4	52.9	1.46
1974	72.1	75.9	53.9	55.3	1.41
1975	72.3	75.9	55.8	57.0	1.36
1976	73.5	76.8	57.7	58.8	1.33
1977	74.1	77.3	59.0	60.1	1.31
1978	74.9	78.2	60.2	61.4	1.30
1979	75.9	79.1	61.6	62.9	1.28
1980	76.3	79.3	62.7	63.8	1.26
1981	76.3	79.4	62.4	63.8	1.27
1982	76.1	79.3	61.5	63.2	1.29
1983	76.2	79.4	61.5	63.4	1.29
1984	76.5	79.6	62.2	64.1	1.28
1985	76.2	79.4	61.8	63.7	1.28
1986	75.9	79.2	61.6	63.7	1.29
1987	76.0	79.4	61.2	63.4	1.30
1988	75.9	79.4	61.1	63.6	1.30

[a]Early prenatal care is defined as care beginning in the first trimester.

SOURCE: Published and unpublished data from the National Center for Health Statistics as reported in Children's Defense Fund (Rosenbaum et al., 1991); additional calculations by the Institute of Medicine.

tent of prenatal care is clearly an important task, and it remains a major challenge for researchers (Culpepper, 1991). For example, where women first receive prenatal care varies according to race. Data from 1982 and 1983, collected during cycle III of the National Survey of Family Growth, show that 80 percent of white women who began prenatal care during the first trimester visited a personal, private physician (as opposed to a hospital, health department, or clinic), whereas only 48 percent of black women receiving early prenatal care did so (National Center for Health Statistics, 1988). Further work is needed to sort out the implications of these and other organizational differences—both in terms of positive and negative consequences.

Recommendations

Improved Data from the Revised Standard Birth Certificate and the 1988 National Maternal and Infant Health Survey. The standard birth cer-

TABLE 3-4　Percentage of Women Receiving Early Prenatal Care,[a] by Race/Ethnicity, 1988

Race/Ethnicity	Percentage
All races	75.9[b]
American Indian	58.1
Black	61.1[b]
Central/South American	63.1
Chinese	82.4
Cuban	83.4
Filipino	78.4
Japanese	86.3
Mexican American	58.3
Puerto Rican	63.3
White	79.4[b]

[a]Early prenatal care is defined as care beginning in the first trimester.
[b]Data received directly from the National Center for Health Statistics' Vital Statistics System.

SOURCE: National Center for Health Statistics (1990c).

tificate has been revised to include more information on risk factors that affect pregnancy. The form now allows check-box entries for each of 16 medical risk factors. More research and analysis are needed to relate prenatal care and birth outcomes to these risk factors.

The 1988 National Maternal and Infant Health Survey (NMIHS; National Center for Health Statistics, 1991) obtained information from mothers, hospitals, and providers on pregnancies, pregnancy outcomes, and early infant health. In addition, a longitudinal follow-up study was begun in 1990. The study will provide more information on the dynamics of prenatal care; child development; and the effects of low birthweight, child nutrition, and exposure to environmental hazards.

The committee supports these efforts and recommends that NCHS expedite the analysis and release of these data. In addition, the committee recommends that research be undertaken to determine the accuracy of birth certificate data through a comparison of those data with data from the NMIHS. Finally, given the importance of financial barriers to access to prenatal care, the committee recommends that the NCHS consider further revision of the birth certificate to include income class and insurance information.

Content and Timing of Prenatal Services. The committee recommends the continuation of research into the measurement of the content of prenatal care, especially for high-risk pregnancies. This research is likely to improve our understanding of the relationship between prenatal care and successful birth outcomes. In this regard the committee supports the National Fetal and Infant Mortality Review Program established by the American College of Obstetrics and Gynecology. This program is designed to assist communities in identifying specific causes of infant and fetal mortality and the barriers that need to be addressed. Community-based studies will also help clarify how the constellation of available resources and the way they are organized affect outcomes.

Financial Barriers to Access. The committee recommends the continuation of efforts to develop a better understanding of the relationship between income and access to prenatal care. The committee was encouraged by the results of a pilot project in New York City that linked birth certificate data with Census Bureau income data by zip code. States should subscribe to the long-term objective of computerizing their birth and death records in ways that will promote small-area analyses and needs assessment—not only in terms of income but also in relation to other characteristics of local communities.

Improved Measurement of Prenatal Services. Although the committee has chosen to use the modified Kessner index as a measure of the adequacy of prenatal care, this method is not without its problems. Federal agencies and the states need to continue to develop better indices of adequate prenatal care. The federal Bureau of Maternal and Child Health, for example, has supported state efforts to develop a common outcome-oriented minimum data set and a standard definition of adequate prenatal care. Efforts should be made to develop an index that measures the timing, sensitivity, content, and quality of prenatal care and that accounts for the effects of various risk factors in determining adequacy.

Outcome Indicator: Infant Mortality

Infant mortality refers to children who die before their first birthday. Subcomponent measures of infant mortality are derived by dividing the first year after birth into two stages: neonatal (28 days old or younger) and postneonatal (between 28 days and 1 year of age). Each measure may provide potentially useful information about barriers to health care access. Dividing the first year of life into two parts allows identification of the most appropriate health interventions for specific infant age groups. Reducing neonatal mortality requires not only that steps be taken during pregnancy to increase birthweight but also that intrapartum and newborn care be improved. To achieve the latter, reorganized perinatal services have been put in place. Interventions intended to reduce postneonatal mortality must focus on improving well- and sick-child care and on intensive follow-up of high-risk infants (Centers for Disease Control, 1989b).

Infant mortality data have been widely collected throughout the world, primarily as a way to assess the success or failure of national health care systems. Infant mortality is a useful, although indirect, indicator of the adequacy of prenatal care and of access to neonatal intensive care units (NICUs) and care in the first year of life. The relationship between inadequate prenatal care and infant mortality has become less precise, however, as NICUs have become more widely available and new therapeutic methods for improving the survivability of premature babies have been developed.

Measuring the Indicator

Infant mortality is expressed as the number of deaths per 1,000 live births. National data on infant deaths are compiled by the NCHS. Unfortunately, most of the routinely available data on infant mortality do not provide information about access barriers, which inhibits our ability to better understand the relationship between financial, structural, and personal barriers and outcomes. To analyze factors that contribute to infant mortality, death certificates frequently are "linked" to birth records, which contain information about the mother's use of prenatal care services and other factors that influence the outcome of pregnancy. As noted previously, the revised birth certificate has space for information on 16 medical risk factors. The new certificate also provides space for physicians to record information on obstetrical procedures, method of delivery, and abnormal conditions of the newborn. This kind of information should make the linking of birth and death certificates of even greater value in understanding the causes of infant mortality.

Trends in the Data

Table 3-5 displays infant mortality rates, by race, for selected years from 1970 to 1990. Rates through 1988 are based on complete records and include information on race. Provisional data for 1989 and 1990 are based on a 10 percent sample of deaths. Given the 1987 and 1988 experiences, those provisional rates are likely to be very close to the actual rates.

Infant death rates in the United States have been halved over the past 20 years, from 20 per 1,000 live births in 1970 to 9.1 per 1,000 live births in 1990. The 1990 rate is about 7 percent lower than the 1989 rate and is the lowest ever for the United States. The greatest improvement was seen for neonatal mortality; the greatest reduction in deaths was seen for respiratory distress syndrome, as a result of improved forms of treatment (National Center for Health Statistics, 1990a).

The 7 percent reduction between 1989 and 1990 was significantly higher than in previous years during the 1980s, when the average yearly decline

TABLE 3-5   Infant Mortality Rates by Race and Black/White Ratios,
Selected Years, 1970–1990

Year	All Races	White	All Nonwhite	Black	Ratio, Black/White
Infant Mortality Rates[a]					
1970	20.0	17.8	30.9	32.6	1.83
1975	16.1	14.2	24.2	26.2	1.84
1980	12.6	11.0	19.1	21.4	1.94
1981	11.9	10.5	17.8	20.0	1.90
1982	11.5	10.1	17.3	19.6	1.94
1983	11.2	9.7	16.8	19.2	1.98
1984	10.8	9.4	16.1	18.4	1.96
1985	10.6	9.3	15.8	18.2	1.96
1986	10.4	8.9	15.7	18.0	2.02
1987	10.1	8.6	15.4	17.9	2.08
1988	10.0	8.5	15.0	17.6	2.07
1989	9.7[b]	N.a.	N.a.	N.a.	
1990	9.1[b]	N.a.	N.a.	N.a.	
Neonatal Mortality Rates[c]					
1970	15.1	13.8	21.4	22.8	1.65
1975	11.6	10.4	16.8	18.3	1.76
1980	8.5	7.5	12.5	14.1	1.88
1981	8.0	7.1	11.8	13.4	1.89
1982	7.7	6.8	11.3	13.1	1.93
1983	7.3	6.4	10.8	12.4	1.94
1984	7.0	6.2	10.2	11.8	1.90
1985	7.0	6.1	10.3	12.1	1.98
1986	6.7	5.8	10.1	11.7	2.02
1987	6.5	5.5	10.0	11.7	2.13
1988	6.3	5.4	9.7	11.5	2.13
1989	6.3[b]	N.a.	N.a.	N.a.	
1990	5.7[b]	N.a.	N.a.	N.a.	
Postneonatal Mortality Rate[d]					
1970	4.9	4.0	9.5	9.9	2.48
1975	4.5	3.8	7.5	7.9	2.08
1980	4.1	3.5	6.6	7.3	2.08
1981	3.9	3.4	6.0	6.6	1.94
1982	3.8	3.3	5.9	6.6	2.00
1983	3.9	3.3	6.0	6.8	2.06
1984	3.8	3.3	5.8	6.5	1.97
1985	3.7	3.2	5.5	6.1	1.90
1986	3.6	3.1	5.6	6.3	2.03
1987	3.6	3.1	5.4	6.1	1.97
1988	3.6	3.1	5.4	6.2	2.00
1989	3.5[b]	N.a.	N.a.	N.a.	
1990	3.3[b]	N.a.	N.a.	N.a.	

TABLE 3-5 *Continued*

N.a., not available.

[a]Deaths before the age of one year.

[b]Provisional infant mortality rates based on a 10 percent sample. The 1987 provisional rate was 10 percent (versus a 10.1 percent final rate). The 1988 provisional rate was 9.9 percent (versus a 10.0 percent final rate).

[c]Deaths at less that 28 days.

[d]Deaths from 28 days to one year of age.

SOURCES: For 1970–1988 data, National Center for Health Statistics (1990a); for 1989–1990 data, National Center for Health Statistics (1990b).

was less than 3 percent. The average rate of decline during the 1980s was well below the 4.7 percent experienced during the 1970s.

As the table shows, the past 20 years have also seen a dramatic decrease in the neonatal mortality rate, from 15.1 per 1,000 live births in 1970 to a provisional 5.7 per 1,000 in 1990. Over the same period, the decline in the postneonatal rate was less striking; it fell from 4.9 percent to a provisional 3.3 percent. During the 1980s, a 28 percent reduction occurred in the overall infant mortality rate, with the greatest decrease (33 percent) arising from improved neonatal mortality rates and the smallest (19 percent) stemming from improvements in postneonatal mortality. The comparable figures for the 1970s were 37 percent, 44 percent, and 16 percent for improvements in overall mortality, neonatal mortality, and postneonatal mortality, respectively.

A striking aspect of infant mortality data is the contrast between the white and black populations. As Table 3-5 shows, infant mortality rates for blacks are much higher than for whites. The absolute differences in rates between the races have narrowed, from approximately 15 more black deaths per 1,000 live births in 1970 to approximately 9 more deaths in 1988; however, the ratio of black to white infant deaths has increased substantially. In 1970 blacks were 85 percent more likely than whites to die during the first year after birth. By 1988 black infants were more than twice as likely as whites to die during their first year. In 1970 blacks were 65 percent more likely than whites to die during the first month after birth; by 1988 they were more than twice as likely to die. In 1975 blacks were twice as likely as whites to die during the postneonatal period, a difference that remained largely unchanged through 1988.

Table 3-6 provides data on infant mortality according to the race or ethnicity of the mother. The data are derived from the linked birth and death records for 1983–1985. Using linked birth and death records addresses the inconsistencies between the information on the two records. Although this information is quite constant for blacks and whites, it can vary

TABLE 3-6 Infant Mortality Rates[a] According to Race/Ethnicity of the Mother, 1983–1985 Birth Cohorts

Race/Ethnicity[b]	Neonatal	Postneonatal	Infant Mortality
American Indian	6.7	7.2	13.9
Black	12.2	6.4	18.7
Central/South American	5.7	2.5	8.2
Chinese	4.3	3.1	7.4
Cuban	5.9	2.2	8.0
Filipino	5.3	2.9	8.2
Japanese	3.4	2.6	6.0
Mexican American	5.7	3.2	8.8
Puerto Rican	8.3	4.0	12.3
White	5.9	3.1	9.0

[a]Deaths per 1,000 live births.
[b]Hispanic data were collected from 23 states and the District of Columbia.

SOURCE: National Center for Health Statistics (1990c).

by as much as 25 to 40 percent for American Indians and for some Asian and Pacific Island groups. For this reason the annual records can be misleading, and conclusions must be drawn with caution.

American Indians and Puerto Ricans (as well as blacks) have infant mortality rates that are well above the national averages. For Puerto Ricans, higher infant mortality rates are a result of both high neonatal and postneonatal mortality rates. The high rate among American Indians is primarily due to the group's higher postneonatal death rate. Unfortunately, more recent data are not currently available (National Center for Health Statistics, 1990a).

The U.S. Department of Health and Human Services' (DHHS) Health Objectives for the Year 2000 set a national target of no more than 7 infant deaths per 1,000 live births for the year 2000 (U.S. Public Health Service, 1991). The target for blacks is 11 deaths per 1,000 births; for American Indians, 8.5 deaths per 1,000 live births; and for Puerto Ricans, 8 deaths per 1,000 live births.

Recommendations

Financial and Insurance Barriers. The committee supports NCHS's plans to continue to link birth and death records but also believes that efforts should be made to add source-of-payment information to both records. In the interim the committee recommends efforts to use zip codes to link information from birth certificates to income information from census data.

Access-Sensitive Measures of Infant Mortality. The problem with infant mortality rates as an indicator of access is that they include causes of death, which at present cannot be affected by the personal health care system. The committee believes that there is a need for additional efforts to determine how best to aggregate the specific *International Classification of Diseases* (9th revision; U.S. Department of Health and Human Services, 1991) categories listed on death certificates into overall classes, which can be categorized as preventable or nonpreventable.

Hispanic Data by Subgroup. The committee encourages NCHS's plans to use the linked birth and infant death files to produce infant death information by specific racial and ethnic subgroups. This proposal is particularly important for Hispanics, whose mortality rates range from well above average for Puerto Ricans to below average for Cubans.

Black–White Gap in Infant Mortality. The committee recommends further research into the contribution of access barriers to the unacceptably large and widening gap in infant mortality between whites and blacks. Particular attention should be focused on the role of financial and insurance barriers as well as the linkage between personal health services and key social services.

Outcome Indicator: Low Birthweight

Infants weighing less than 2,500 grams (5.5 pounds) are considered to be of low birthweight. Very-low-birthweight infants, weigh less than 1,500 grams (3.3 pounds) at birth.

The most important predictor of infant survival is birthweight; survival improves exponentially as birthweight increases to its optimum level (Centers for Disease Control, 1989b). However, a successful birth is one that not only produces a live baby but also a healthy one. Compared with infants weighing more than 2,500 grams, low-birthweight and very-low-birthweight babies are much more likely to die during the first year of life and to be hospitalized more frequently. They also have a higher incidence of acute infections and suffer from a range of developmental, behavioral, and physical disabilities. Births of low-birthweight and very-low-birthweight infants frequently are associated with inadequate prenatal care and lack of access to nutrition services. Unlike infant mortality (which may be influenced both by the health care services received by the mother during pregnancy and the care received by the infant up to one year after delivery), low birthweight and very low birthweight are outcome indicators specific to the services that the mother received prior to giving birth.

Measuring the Indicator

Low birthweight and very low birthweight are expressed as the percentage of live births weighing less than 2,500 grams and 1,500 grams, respectively. The major source of data on low birthweight and very low birthweight is the birth certificate. Information from birth records is sent by the states to NCHS. The 1988 NMIHS (National Center for Health Statistics, 1991) provides more detailed information about the extent of prenatal care and risk factors associated with low birthweight and very low birthweight.

Additional understanding of the low-birthweight problem should be possible when 1989 birth certificate data become available for analysis. The revised birth certificate includes information on medical risk factors and maternal behavior during pregnancy (tobacco and alcohol use) as well as low maternal weight gain—all factors that have been associated with low birthweight.

Efforts to monitor changes in low birthweight are hindered by the considerable time lag between data collection and publication. Similar delays are present in the availability of national linked birth and death certificate data, which are the best source for determining the relationship between low birthweight and poor health outcomes (Miller et al., 1989). In addition, as is true for all events dependent on birth records, no data are available on the source of payment for care.

Trends in the Data

Table 3-7 displays the percentage of infants of low birthweight by race in the United States for selected years from 1970 through 1988, the last year for which data are available. What is most striking is how little change there has been over time. Although there was some decline in low-birthweight births during the 1970s, no improvement was apparent during the 1980s. The percentage of low-birthweight black infants also deserves note. The ratio of black to white low-birthweight births in 1970 was 2.04. A slow but steady increase in the disparity has occurred over the past 20 years, until by 1988 the ratio reached 2.32. The percentage of low-birthweight babies born to nonwhites in 1988 was the same as in 1976. Table 3-8 shows low-birthweight births for 1988 by racial and ethnic groups. Unlike the previous table, these data are based on the race/ethnicity of the mother rather than the infant.

Table 3-8 reveals the heterogeneity of the Hispanic population. The percentage of low-birthweight infants varies from 5.6 per 1,000 live births for Mexican American and Central and South American women to 9.4 per 1,000 live births for Puerto Rican women. The incidence of low birthweight among Puerto Ricans was approximately two-thirds higher than that of white women.

TABLE 3-7 Percentage of Low-Birthweight Infants, by Race, Selected Years, 1970–1988

Year	All Races	All White	Nonwhite	Black	Ratio, Black/White
1970	7.9	6.8	13.9	13.3	2.04
1971	7.7	6.6	13.4	12.7	2.03
1972	7.7	6.5	13.6	12.9	2.09
1973	7.6	6.4	13.3	12.5	2.08
1974	7.4	6.3	13.1	12.4	2.08
1975	7.4	6.3	13.1	12.2	2.08
1976	7.3	6.1	13.0	12.1	2.13
1977	7.1	5.9	12.8	11.9	2.17
1978	7.1	5.9	12.8	11.9	2.17
1979	6.9	5.8	12.6	11.6	2.17
1980	6.8	5.7	12.5	11.5	2.19
1981	6.8	5.7	12.5	11.4	2.19
1982	6.8	5.6	12.4	11.2	2.21
1983	6.8	5.6	12.6	11.2	2.25
1984	6.7	5.6	12.4	11.1	2.21
1985	6.8	5.6	12.4	11.1	2.21
1986	6.8	5.6	12.5	11.2	2.23
1987	6.9	5.7	12.7	11.3	2.23
1988	6.9	5.6	13.0	11.5	2.32

SOURCE: Rosenbaum et al. (1991).

The national picture is even less encouraging for very-low-birthweight babies. This indicator has shown little change, increasing from 1.15 percent of total births in 1979 to 1.24 percent of the total in 1988 (Rosenbaum et al., 1991). Among blacks the rate rose from 2.37 percent in 1979 to 2.78 percent in 1988.[1] In 1988 black women were three times as likely as white women to have a very-low-birthweight baby, and Puerto Rican women were about 80 percent more likely. Other racial and ethnic groups had approximately the same risk of having a very-low-birthweight infant as whites (National Center for Health Statistics, 1990a).

The DHHS's Health Objectives for the Year 2000 set a goal of reducing the incidence of low birthweight to 5 per 1,000 live births, the same rate proposed in the department's health plan for 1990 (U.S. Public Health Service, 1991). For very-low-birthweight infants, the Year 2000 goal is 1 per

---

[1]Increasingly, such interventions as early delivery of a fetus at risk of in utero death result in the birth of very-low-birthweight infants. Whether this is occurring in sufficiently large numbers to alter national statistical trends is unclear. The extent to which comparison between blacks and whites is influenced by differences in the rate of this intervention is also unclear.

TABLE 3-8   Percentage of Low-Birthweight
Infants by Race/Ethnicity of Mother, 1988

Race/Ethnicity[a]	Percentage
American Indian	6.0
Black	13.3
Central/South American	5.6
Chinese	4.6
Cuban	5.9
Filipino	7.1
Japanese	6.7
Mexican American	5.6
Puerto Rican	9.4
White	5.7

[a]Hispanic data were collected from 30 states and the
District of Columbia.

SOURCE: National Center for Health Statistics (1990b).

100 live births. The Year 2000 objectives set a separate target for blacks of
9 for low birthweight and 2 for very low birthweight. Blacks were the only
racial or ethnic group that failed to meet the department's 1990 goal of
reducing the low birthweight rate to 9 percent or less.

To understand access barriers that are likely to contribute to the incidence of low birthweight, it is helpful to begin with the known correlates.
A variety of factors are correlated with low birthweight and very low birthweight; they have been divided into several categories, including demographic characteristics, medical risks before and during the current pregnancy, and behavioral and environmental risks (Institute of Medicine, 1985).
Demographic characteristics that may predispose an infant to low birthweight include low socioeconomic status, limited formal education, bearing
children either at a young age (under 17) or an older age (over 34), and
being unmarried.   Medical risks include such factors as poor obstetrical
history, certain diseases and conditions, poor nutritional status, poor weight
gain, and short interpregnancy interval. Behavioral and environmental risks
include personal behaviors such as smoking, alcohol and drug abuse, and
environmental exposure to toxic substances. Also counted under this rubric
is inadequate or no prenatal care.

A significant amount of research attention has focused on whether the
disparity in the rates of low birthweight between whites and blacks can be
explained solely by differences in access barriers and maternal risk factors.
The manner in which birthweight data have been analyzed seems to indicate
that low birthweight is significantly related to race.   However, whether

race, per se, is causally related to low birthweight or whether it is a proxy for differences in medical access and socioeconomic status is a matter currently under debate. By controlling for factors other than race, at least one study has shown that the higher rates of prematurity (a birth outcome closely linked to low birthweight) experienced by blacks are attributable to specific medical and socioeconomic characteristics rather than race (Lieberman et al., 1987). These results, however, must be confirmed by other studies with larger samples (Behrman, 1987).

Recommendations

Racial and Ethnic Differences in Low Birthweight. The committee believes that research and analysis should focus on determining the reasons for the large, persistent, and apparently increasing differences in the incidence of low birthweight and very low birthweight among blacks and other racial and ethnic minority groups. It is important that these efforts identify how various barriers affect access to care and that they determine the impact of medical risk factors and socioeconomic factors. It is hoped that data from the revised birth certificate and the 1988 NMIHS (and its 1990 follow-up) will provide greater understanding of this most significant problem.

Financial Barriers. The committee believes that the effects on low birthweight of insurance status and income need to be examined in greater detail. Analyses that use data from the NMIHS or, if available, comparisons of selected states that have linked Medicaid and birth certificate data could provide useful information about the impact of insurance coverage. Data on maternal income may come out of efforts to link zip code data to income information from the Census Bureau.

Delays in Data Availability. There have been concerns that the time lag between data collection and publication of NCHS findings is unnecessarily long and that this lag significantly interferes with the ability to plan, implement, and evaluate public policies. The committee recommends that the Public Health Service investigate these complaints and determine whether efforts to improve the timeliness of NCHS reports are warranted. Consideration should be given to publishing NCHS data as they are received, on a rolling, monthly basis.

Impact of Culture. Recent analysis of the Hispanic Health and Nutrition Examination Survey shows that first-generation Mexican American women have better low-birthweight experiences than those born in the United States (Scribner and Dwyer, 1989). The opposite has been shown to be true for Southeast Asian immigrants (Li et al., 1990). It is as yet unclear whether cultural factors, underreporting of deaths, or other factors may be governing these outcomes. Further research on this topic is warranted.

Outcome Indicator: Congenital Syphilis

Syphilis is a chronic contagious disease caused by a spirochete of *Treponema palladium*, a bacterium. In adults the disease goes through three stages: the development of skin lesions (primary syphilis); the spread, within two to six months, of lesions into the organs and tissues (secondary syphilis); and the development of skin ulcers and tumors, often with involvement of the skeletal, cardiovascular, and nervous systems (tertiary syphilis). Infants can develop congenital syphilis if infected by their mother during pregnancy or at the time of delivery. Although syphilis may cause rapid onset of severe illness or death in infants (up to 40 percent), the disease responds well to treatment with penicillin.

Each case of congenital syphilis indicates either a lack of any prenatal care (even one prenatal care visit should alert the health care provider to the need for treatment) or a lack of adequate care (a prenatal visit at which an infected mother is not diagnosed is inadequate). In most cases, treatment of syphilis at least 30 days prior to delivery should prevent infection in the infant.

A 1990 editorial in the *American Journal of Public Health* had this comment:

> Congenital syphilis should be a disease of the past. It is fully preventable by treating infected women with penicillin early in pregnancy, provided that infection or reinfection late in pregnancy does not occur. It is therefore a sentinel health condition: its occurrence marks the failure of both the syphilis control program and the prenatal care system.

The recent rise in rates of congenital syphilis in certain geographic areas of the United States is thought to be due in part to the increase in cocaine use (particularly "crack" cocaine), with its attendant transmission of sexually transmitted diseases. Rates of congenital syphilis, therefore, may also indicate a lack of available, acceptable drug treatment services for pregnant women.

Measuring the Indicator

The incidence of congenital syphilis is measured in numbers of cases per 100,000 population. The presence of the condition can be determined by one of several serologic tests. Test results are reported by physicians to their state health departments, which then forward the results to the Centers for Disease Control (CDC).

The change in 1988 of CDC's case definition for reporting congenital syphilis makes it difficult to interpret changes in the data before that year. The new definition broadened and simplified the reporting criteria. The earlier, more complex reporting requirements depended on extensive physical and laboratory findings at birth and during subsequent follow-up visits. They did not call for including stillborn fetuses with the disease in the overall tally of syphilis incidence.

The new definition is certain to result in an increase in reported cases of congenital syphilis during the short transition period between use of the old and use of the new definition. In one study, based on cases reported in Los Angeles County in 1987, the new definition resulted in a fivefold increase in cases, from 39 to 205 (Cohen et al., 1990).

Counterbalancing the increase in rates expected under the new CDC case definition is the belief that the incidence of congenital syphilis may be underreported because of the failure of physicians to diagnose the disease. In some instances, serologic tests may fail to detect infection in an infant at the time of birth. This may be because the child, although infected, has not yet produced syphilis antibodies on which the test relies for a positive result. The diagnosis of congenital syphilis may also be missed if only the mother is tested (Cohen, 1991). Even when both mother and infant test negative for syphilis at delivery, infection cannot be ruled out because a mother's acquisition of syphilis late in pregnancy may not be detected (Dorfman and Glaser, 1990).

Trends in the Data

Table 3-9 displays the total number of cases of syphilis and cases per 100,000 population for both adult (primary and secondary) and congenital syphilis for selected years from 1970 through 1990. Information on both primary and secondary syphilis is included because the incidence of congenital syphilis closely mirrors the rate of primary and secondary infection in women and because treatment of infected women is the only way to prevent congenital syphilis. The relationship appears graphically in Figure 3-1, which shows the yearly cases of congenital syphilis and the rate of primary and secondary syphilis in women and in men.

The incidence of primary and secondary syphilis in the United States declined from 16.73 per 100,000 in 1950 to 11.45 cases per 100,000 in 1985. It increased steadily through 1990, however, when it reached 20.10, the highest level in the past 40 years.

There are marked differences in the incidence of syphilis among whites, blacks, and other racial and ethnic groups in the United States. Although the incidence for both whites and blacks fell between 1982 and 1985, in 1986 the rates for blacks began to increase. Between 1985 and 1989 the

TABLE 3-9   Disease Rates for Primary, Secondary, and Congenital
Syphilis, Selected Years, 1970–1990

| | Adult Syphilis, Primary and Secondary | | | | | |
| | Men and Women | | Women Only | | Congenital Syphilis | |
Year	No. of Cases	Cases/ 100,000 Population	No. of Cases	Cases/ 100,000 Population	No. of Cases	Cases/ 100,000 Population
1970	21,982	10.89	N.a.	N.a.	1,953	0.97
1980	27,204	12.06	N.a.	N.a.	277	0.12
1985	27,131	11.45	N.a.	N.a.	329	0.14
1986	27,883	11.65	9,197	7.5	410	0.17
1987	35,147	14.54	13,257	10.6	681	0.28
1988	40,117	16.43	16,172	12.9	751	0.30
1989	44,540	18.07	19,047	15.0	941	0.38
1990	50,223	20.10	22,106	17.3	2,899	1.16

N.a., not available.

SOURCES: National Center for Health Statistics (1990c); Centers for Disease Control data.

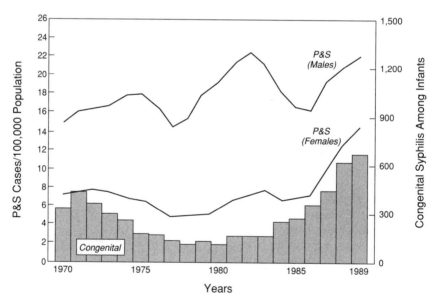

FIGURE 3-1   Cases of congenital syphilis among infants under one year of age
and cases of primary and secondary syphilis (P&S) per 100,000 population, by sex,
1970–1989. SOURCE: Centers for Disease Control (1989c).

rate for blacks increased by 132 percent, from 52.6 to 121.8 cases per 100,000 population. It more than doubled in 22 states and the District of Columbia and rose more than fourfold in 10 states. Between 1981 and 1989 the black-to-white incidence rate ratio increased from 14.5 to 47.8. Incidence rates for Asian Americans and Pacific Islanders paralleled those for whites through 1989, whereas the rates for Hispanics remained between the rates for whites and blacks (Rolfs and Nakashima, 1990).

A number of studies have linked the spread of syphilis to increased drug use, particularly cocaine, which often is tied to drug-related high-risk sexual behaviors such as prostitution (Fullilove et al., 1990; McLaughlin et al., 1989; Schwarcz et al., 1989). It also appears that drug use is directly associated with low levels of prenatal care utilization. One study of mothers infected with syphilis who also used cocaine found that 75.8 percent had received no prenatal care (Nanda et al., 1990).

The Year 2000 Health Objective for primary and secondary syphilis in adults is 10 per 100,000 population. For blacks a separate goal is laid out: 65 per 100,000 population. The reasons for the extreme disparity between syphilis incidence rates for blacks and whites are unclear.

Recommendations

Black–White Disparities. The committee recommends that additional research and analyses be conducted to better understand the large disparity between the incidence of primary and secondary syphilis for blacks and whites. Particular emphasis should be placed on the role of barriers to access to health care services.

Drug Use and Prenatal Care Services. The committee also believes that research should be conducted to examine the relationships among drug use, sexually transmitted diseases, and the use of prenatal care services. Such research may shed light on ways of making prenatal care and substance abuse treatment more accessible to this extremely high-risk population and lead to better measures of structural barriers to access.

OBJECTIVE 2: REDUCING THE INCIDENCE OF VACCINE-PREVENTABLE CHILDHOOD DISEASES

Utilization Indicator: Preschool Immunization

Immunization provides protection from infectious diseases, including some that are potentially life threatening. Generally, a vaccine is made up of key parts of a disease organism, or the entire organism is modified so as not to cause disease. Once introduced into the human body, the vaccine stimulates the production of antibodies and lymphocytes capable of recognizing and destroying the disease-causing microbe.

The immunization of children against polio, measles, mumps, rubella, diphtheria, pertussis, and tetanus has gained wide acceptance in the United States and other countries, both as a means for providing protection to individuals and as a public health measure. (*Haemophilus influenzae* type b [HIB] encephalitis immunization, while also important, has not been recommended for a sufficient period of time for data to be available.) Routine immunization schedules for children are shown in Table 3-10.

When carried out on a wide scale, immunization programs can dramatically reduce the incidence of certain childhood diseases. Immunization carried out incompletely or only in select population groups, however, can result in higher rates of preventable illness and death than would be expected with more complete vaccine coverage. There is an acknowledged public-private responsibility for immunizing children in the United States. For school-age children, vaccination is required by law in most jurisdictions, but it is generally not required for younger children. Low rates of immunization may indicate the presence of important barriers to other preventive health care services as well. Although nearly all children are vaccinated by the time they begin school (because of statutory requirements), the key access question is whether children are being immunized in accordance with recommended schedules, which require the first immunization at 2 months of age.

Measuring the Indicator

Immunization rates are expressed as the percentage of preschool-age children (ages 1–4) who have been vaccinated. Rates are reported by disease for purposes of access monitoring.

A major problem with state and national efforts to vaccinate children against disease is that there is currently no ongoing routine method of monitoring immunization levels of preschool children. The national immunization survey has not been conducted since 1985; thus, our nationwide estimates are increasingly out of date. Even the accuracy of data obtained in this type of survey is questionable because survey respondents are often expected to recall specific events that happened many years before. This task is made doubly difficult if respondents have more than one child.

Trends in the Data

Table 3-11 displays unpublished survey data on vaccination rates for U.S. children ages 1–4 for selected years from 1970 to 1985. In 1985 the immunization rates ranged from 55.3 percent for polio to 64.9 percent for

TABLE 3-10   Recommended Immunization Schedule for Children

Age	Vaccines
2 Months	DPT^a (first) TOPV^b (first)
4 Months	DPT (second) TOPV (second)
6 Months	DPT (third)
15 Months	Measles^c Mumps^c Rubella^c DPT (fourth) TOPV (third)
18 Months	HIB conjugate^d
At school entry (4–6 Years)	MMR, DPT (fifth) TOPV (fourth)

^{a}DPT, diphtheria and pertussis and tetanus toxoids vaccine adsorbed; five doses recommended.

^{b}TOPV, trivalent oral polio vaccine (live); four doses recommended; however, some physicians may elect to give one additional dose at 6 months of age.

^{c}May be combined as a single injection vaccine (MMR).

^{d}*Haemophilus influenzae* type b conjugate vaccine.

SOURCE: Hinman (1990).

DPT. The survey indicated declines in vaccination levels of DPT and polio since 1970 and some variation but no clear trends in vaccination rates for the other diseases (particularly during 1983–1985). The same general patterns apply when one considers vaccination by race and by place of residence (inside or outside a metropolitan statistical area, or MSA). However, whites were much more likely to have been vaccinated than children of other races. In addition, beginning in 1976, the survey found that children in the central-city portion of an MSA were less likely to be vaccinated than children in other MSA areas, including the suburbs, or those living outside the MSA altogether.

Even taking into account the possibility of some underreporting, U.S. vaccination rates for children are well below those in some European countries. For example, in 1987 in Denmark, West Germany, and the Netherlands, and in 1986 in France, polio immunization levels among children

TABLE 3-11   Vaccinations of Children 1–4 Years of Age (as percentage of population) for Selected Diseases, by Race and Residence in Metropolitan Statistical Area (MSA), 1970, 1976, and 1983–1985

Vaccination and Year	Total	Race		Inside MSA		Outside MSA
		White	All Other	Central City	Remaining Areas	Outside MSA
DPT[a,b]						
1970	76.1	79.7	58.8	68.9	80.7	77.1
1976	71.4	75.3	53.2	64.1	75.7	72.9
1983	65.7	70.1	47.7	55.4	69.4	69.4
1984	65.7	69.1	51.3	57.9	66.6	69.8
1985	64.9	68.7	48.7	55.5	68.4	67.9
Measles						
1970	57.2	60.4	41.9	55.2	61.7	54.3
1976	65.9	68.3	54.8	62.5	67.2	67.3
1983	64.9	66.8	57.2	60.4	66.3	66.7
1984	62.8	65.4	52.0	56.6	63.3	66.4
1985	60.8	63.6	48.8	55.5	63.3	61.9
Mumps						
1970	N.a.	N.a.	N.a.	N.a.	N.a.	N.a.
1976	48.3	50.3	38.7	45.6	50.7	47.9
1983	59.5	61.8	50.0	52.6	60.2	63.6
1984	58.7	61.3	47.7	51.8	58.3	63.6
1985	58.9	61.8	47.0	52.4	61.0	61.4
Polio[b]						
1970	65.9	69.2	50.1	61.0	70.8	64.7
1976	61.6	66.2	39.9	53.8	65.3	63.9
1983	57.0	61.9	36.7	47.7	60.3	60.3
1984	54.8	58.4	39.9	48.7	55.2	58.5
1985	55.3	58.9	40.1	47.1	58.4	58.0
Rubella						
1970	37.2	38.3	31.8	38.3	39.2	34.3
1976	61.7	63.8	51.5	59.5	63.5	61.5
1983	64.0	66.3	54.7	59.5	65.2	66.0
1984	60.9	63.9	48.3	56.1	60.4	64.6
1985	58.9	61.6	47.7	53.9	61.0	60.3
Respondents consulting vaccination records, 1985[c]						
DPT[a,b]	87.0	88.5	75.2	79.6	89.7	88.6
Measles	76.9	78.1	67.2	73.5	76.7	79.0
Mumps	75.5	77.1	62.7	70.5	76.8	77.0
Polio[b]	75.7	77.5	61.5	68.9	79.6	75.9
Rubella	73.8	75.0	64.1	70.4	75.0	74.6

TABLE 3-11 *Continued*

N.a., not available.

NOTE: Beginning in 1976 the category "don't know" was added to response categories. Prior to 1976 the lack of this option resulted in some forced positive answers, particularly for vaccinations requiring multiple-dose schedules, that is, polio and DPT.

[a]Diphtheria-pertussis-tetanus.

[b]Three doses or more.

[c]The data in this panel are based only on 35 percent of white respondents and 19 percent of all other respondents who consulted records for some or all vaccination questions. One month prior to the interview, all sampled households were asked to check vaccination records, such as those from a private physician, health department, or military.

SOURCE: Unpublished data from the U.S. Immunization Survey, conducted by the Centers for Disease Control, Center for Prevention Services, Division of Immunization.

3 years old or younger exceeded 95 percent. The same success rate was achieved by France, West Germany, and the Netherlands with the DPT vaccine (Williams, 1990). The DHHS in its Health Objectives for the Year 2000 (U.S. Public Health Service, 1991) adopted a goal of immunization for 90 percent of U.S. preschoolers.

Immunization levels for children between the ages of 5 and 6 are significantly higher than those for preschoolers. The reason is that laws in every state require up-to-date vaccinations as a prerequisite to school entry. Provisional data for the 1989–1990 school year indicate that at least 97 percent of students in kindergarten through first grade had received a full course of DPT, polio, and measles-mumps-rubella vaccines (Hinman, 1991). The rates for younger children enrolled in day care centers (95 percent for all vaccines) and Head Start programs (between 94 and 97 percent for all vaccines) were slightly lower. For school-age children and children in day care who must meet the vaccination requirements, the DHHS's Year 2000 Health Objective of at least 95 percent coverage for the basic immunization series has been achieved.

A major barrier to vaccination is financial in that private-sector administration of vaccines currently costs about $300 ($200 for vaccines and $100 for physician visits) before children can enter school. Public-sector prices for the vaccines are approximately $90 (Hinman, 1991). Because parents generally are not charged the full cost of the vaccines, federal support and state willingness to appropriate funds for vaccination have been the deciding factors in whether health departments and nonprofit agencies can vaccinate all those needing the service.

A 1986 survey of health care accessibility found that children of the poor and the near poor were 50 percent more likely than those of higher income groups not to have up-to-date immunizations. The survey found that lack of insurance was even more of a barrier. Only 1 percent and 6 percent of children with Medicaid or private insurance, respectively, lacked up-to-date immunization, compared with 19 percent of those not insured (Wood et al., 1990). Medicaid covers immunizations, either on its own or through its Early Periodic Screening, Diagnosis, and Treatment program; some but not all private insurers offer this coverage. These findings thus show the importance of health insurance coverage for specific services.

In addition to these economic barriers, a number of organizational and structural impediments lie in the way of access to immunization. Key among them is the lack of a comprehensive system in the United States for identifying and notifying individuals who need immunization. Health care providers, for various reasons, may fail to administer all indicated vaccines at a single visit. The process of seeking immunizations itself may contain disincentives if, for example, vaccination is conducted on an appointment-only basis or at times that are inconvenient. Finally, physicians who insist on performing vaccinations only during well-child visits (a laudable goal) may as a result delay immunization for weeks or months, given the backlog of such appointments in many medical offices (Hinman, 1991). In fact, pediatricians and family physicians appear to be more and more reluctant to provide immunizations in the office setting. A survey in Dallas, Texas, found that an increasing number of patients were being referred to public facilities. The reasons included inability of patients to pay, the cost of vaccines to physicians, and, in the case of family practitioners, concern over liability (Schulte et al., 1991).

Recommendations

Immunization Surveys. The CDC has addressed the lack of current data on preschool immunization by adding items to the 1991 National Health Interview Survey and by sponsoring a program of research and demonstration projects targeting specific barriers to immunization. While these activities will fill the immediate need for better insight into immunization status, the committee believes that a long-term solution, based on compiled immunization records (see the next recommendation), will provide more reliable data for the future.

School-Based Reporting System. In most, if not all, school systems, parents are required to submit immunization records prior to enrolling their children. These records contain the dates of specific immunizations, which could be reported to state health departments (and, in turn, to the CDC) in a standard format. This reporting would permit a retrospective analysis of whether the school-age cohort received scheduled vaccinations on time. Consideration should be given to the extent of the burden of including additional information such as place of immunization. The committee recognizes that there may be some drawbacks to the approach in terms of additional paperwork, delayed reporting, and difficulty in linking the data to other types of information that can be obtained through surveys. Nevertheless, the committee believes that the potential of this strategy for improving the accuracy of vaccination reporting is substantial.

Research on Special Populations. Research is needed to understand particular problems in determining the immunization status of special populations (e.g., undocumented aliens) and how barriers discourage specific groups from receiving necessary immunizations.

Outcome Indicator: Incidence of Vaccine-Preventable Childhood Diseases

Measles, mumps, rubella, diphtheria, pertussis, polio, and tetanus are among the most preventable of infectious diseases. (HIB encephalitis immunization, which recently became available, will be recommended for future monitoring.) Although the incidence of these diseases in the United States is low (because of widespread immunization), periodic outbreaks occur because of lapses in immunization coverage. In countries in which effective vaccines are not routinely available, these diseases still cause significant levels of illness and death.

Some countries monitor the immunization status of all age groups. In the United States, however, only the immunization status of entering school-age children is routinely monitored. Although a large percentage of children are vaccinated by the time they begin school, preschool children (under age 5) and immigrants often are not immunized. Inadequate levels of vaccination in these two groups are believed to contribute to outbreaks of vaccine-preventable diseases. Absent a system for monitoring the immunization status of the entire U.S. population, the incidence of vaccine-preventable diseases is a good indicator of access problems related to vaccination, a key preventive health service.

Measuring the Indicator

States report data on the seven selected vaccine-preventable diseases noted above to the CDC, which has developed a set of standardized case definitions for notifiable diseases (Chorba et al., 1990). Incidence can be expressed both as the total number of cases and as cases per 100,000 population. Data are normally collected by month and year; outbreaks of infectious disease, however, typically occur in cycles, once every several years. A low rate of disease in a given year does not indicate the absence of a problem; rather, the disease's magnitude must be interpreted in relation to its natural history. This makes year-to-year comparisons of the number of cases of a particular disease problematic, because a small number of cases in one year may mask a problem with immunization rates.

Any outbreak is an indication of a problem in immunization. Comparing the number of outbreaks, their duration, and the total number of people infected over the course of the outbreak provides the most useful information. To prevent an outbreak, enough people in a given population must be immunized to establish what is termed "herd immunity." An outbreak means that the level of immunity—and thus the level of immunization—in the population is below a certain minimum rate.

A major problem in tracking incidence accurately is that reporting for many of these diseases is incomplete. For diseases that are now rare, non-reporting may occur as a result of incorrect diagnosis. During an outbreak of a disease, individual physicians may become lax in their reporting as more cases surface. This latter problem tends to obscure the magnitude of an outbreak. The current infectious disease reporting system is particularly unreliable for data on the incidence of diseases in special populations. The accuracy of information about incidence among minorities, for example, is influenced by variations in the reporting systems of different states and by variations in the quality and completeness of reporting, which may reflect differences in access to medical care (Buehler et al., 1989).

Trends in the Data

Table 3-12 provides data on the occurrence of the seven vaccine-preventable diseases from 1980 through 1989. The number of cases of diphtheria and paralytic polio was quite small throughout the decade. (The return of these diseases would be a serious sentinel event.) The number of cases of tetanus dropped from 95 in 1980 to 53 in 1989; the number of cases of rubella fell from nearly 4,000 in 1980 to around 400 in 1989. The number of cases of mumps declined from approximately 8,600 in 1980 to below 3,000 in 1985 but then increased in succeeding years, sometimes dramatically. Cases of measles declined substantially in the early 1980s, from 13,500 in 1980 to fewer than 3,000 annually from 1982 through 1985. Measles cases increased to more than 6,000 in 1986; however, after subsiding in 1987 and 1988, measles cases rose to approximately 18,000 in 1989.

The incidence of measles increased more than fivefold from 1988 to 1989, from 1.38 cases per 100,000 to 7.33 per 100,000. The current outbreak saw another escalation in 1990, when more than 25,000 cases were detected. (The actual number may be even higher because it is possible that, as cases of measles became more common, medical facilities became less likely to report them.) The outbreak has focused renewed attention on

TABLE 3-12 Reported Cases of Vaccine-Preventable Diseases, Selected Years, 1970–1989

Year	Diphtheria No. of Cases	Diphtheria Cases/ 100,000	Measles No. of Cases	Measles Cases/ 100,000	Mumps No. of Cases	Mumps Cases/ 100,000	Pertussis No. of Cases	Pertussis Cases/ 100,000	Polio No. of Cases	Polio Cases/ 100,000	Rubella No. of Cases	Rubella Cases/ 100,000	Tetanus No. of Cases	Tetanus Cases/ 100,000
1970	435	0.21	47,351	23.23	104,953	5.55	4,249	2.08	31	0.02	56,552	27.75	109	0.06
1975	307	0.14	24,379	11.44	59,647	27.99	4,249	2.08	31	0.02	16,652	7.81	252	0.12
1980	3	0.0	13,506	5.96	8,576	3.86	1,730	0.82	8	0.00	3,904	1.72	95	0.04
1981	5	0.0	3,124	1.36	4,941	2.20	1,248	0.54	6	0.00	2,077	0.91	72	0.03
1982	2	0.0	1,714	0.74	5,270	2.46	1,895	0.82	8	0.00	2,325	1.00	88	0.04
1983	5	0.0	1,497	0.64	3,355	1.55	2,463	1.05	15	0.01	970	0.41	91	0.04
1984	1	0.0	2,587	1.10	3,021	1.32	2,276	0.96	8	0.00	752	0.32	74	0.03
1985	3	0.0	2,822	1.18	2,982	1.30	3,589	1.50	7	0.00	630	0.26	83	0.03
1986	—	0.0	6,282	1.61	7,790	3.37	4,195	1.74	6	0.00	551	0.23	64	0.03
1987	3	0.0	3,655	1.50	12,848	5.43	2,823	1.16	6	0.00	306	0.13	48	0.02
1988	2	0.0	3,396	1.38	4,866	2.05	3,450	1.40	9	0.00	396	0.16	53	0.02
1989	3	0.0	18,193	7.33	5,712	2.34	4,157	1.67	5	0.00	396	0.16	53	0.02

SOURCE: Centers for Disease Control (1989c).

the problem of inadequate vaccine coverage among young children, particularly minority children and children living in inner cities (National Vaccine Advisory Committee, 1991).

Although the increase in measles cases should serve as a warning of the need for early and widespread immunization, it should not obscure the major progress that has been made in reducing the incidence of this and other vaccine-preventable diseases over the past several decades. There were 435 cases of diphtheria, 47,351 cases of measles, nearly 105,000 cases of mumps, 56,552 cases of rubella, and 109 cases of tetanus in 1970. Only cases of pertussis, after declining for most of the 1970s and 1980s, have risen to a level comparable to that in 1970.

The DHHS's Health Objectives for the Year 2000 propose the eradication of diphtheria and tetanus (in the under-25 age group) and all cases of polio, measles, and rubella. For mumps the Year 2000 goal is 500 cases; for pertussis it is 1,000 cases.

Case reporting of preventable childhood diseases among racial and ethnic minorities is largely incomplete. In one study approximately 40 percent of case reports did not specify the race or ethnicity of the patient. Existing data indicate that minority children, compared with white children, exhibit higher rates of infectious diseases during an epidemic. For example, in 1987 the incidence of measles among Hispanics (2.24 per 100,000 population) was four to five times higher than for other groups (Buehler et al., 1989). The reporting of information about insurance status, family income, and other barriers to access also is incomplete. Moreover, if it is true, as some believe, that private physicians are increasingly reluctant to give immunizations, the site of immunization will be an additional important clue to the barriers that may need to be overcome.

Recommendations

Increased Surveillance. The committee recommends that disease surveillance activities be increased to monitor outbreaks of infectious disease. The data gathered by such efforts should be used to determine whether higher-than-expected rates of preventable diseases are due to identifiable access-related problems. For example, outbreaks provide an opportunity to understand in greater depth how financial and structural barriers faced by vulnerable populations interfere with their ability to obtain preventive services, including immunization.

Provider Education. The committee recommends that CDC intensify its efforts to alert physicians and local health agencies to the importance of reporting cases of infectious diseases. To that end, CDC surveillance activities should be strengthened.

OBJECTIVE 3: EARLY DETECTION AND DIAGNOSIS
OF TREATABLE DISEASES

Utilization Indicators: Breast and Cervical
Cancer Screening Procedures

There are a number of diseases for which early detection is important enough to justify screening large segments of the population. For the screening to be worthwhile, an effective medical intervention must be available that can treat the disease of interest at an early stage. (However, not all of the screening tests that are justified in clinical practice are useful as access indicators.)

Two sets of screening tests—clinical breast examinations (physical palpation by a health care professional) and mammography for detecting breast cancer, and Pap smears for detecting cervical dysplasia and the less commonly occurring invasive cervical carcinoma—have high sensitivity and high yield; they also detect conditions with high prevalence. Moreover, morbidity and mortality from these cancers are reduced when they are detected at an early stage and the patient is treated appropriately. The timing of the screening tests depends on the age and risk profile of the woman being tested. In most cases the earlier in its progression that the disease is detected, the greater the chance of preventing cancer-related mortality.

For some women less than optimal use of these screening tests indicates the presence of one or more barriers to primary health care services. Yet for other women the failure to undergo a recommended screening test may reflect a lack of knowledge about the test's benefits or insufficient counseling by the woman's health care provider. These latter circumstances are less clearly a problem of access to health care than an indication of poor quality or inadequate medical care. If specific groups consistently receive substandard care, however, this could indicate the presence of an access barrier.

Measuring the Indicator

The measure of utilization of breast cancer and cervical cancer screening tests is the percentage of women in specific age groups who undergo the procedures during a given time period. Two of the primary sources of data for monitoring the use of cancer screening services are the National Health Interview Survey (NHIS), conducted periodically by the National Center for Health Statistics, and the Behavioral Risk Factor Surveillance System, a state-based program of periodic surveys sponsored by the CDC. The most recent data on mammography come from a special survey completed in 1990, the Mammography Attitudes and Usage Study.

Because Objective 3 focuses on routine preventive screening services, we report data from the NHIS that distinguish screening procedures from the same tests that are also ordered for patients who require diagnostic workups as a follow-up to specific health problems. In interpreting trend data it is important to determine whether the data include both categories of patients. Because there has been special interest in the effects of language and culture on the use of screening services, the NHIS breaks out data for Hispanics.

One problem of interpreting data on the use of screening services is the difficulties involved in separating medical access problems from concerns about the quality or adequacy of the medical care itself. It may be that access to screening services is tied in complex ways to the structural characteristics of the delivery system, aspects that have not been investigated by researchers. Some of the difficulty in distinguishing true access problems from other influences on screening behavior may be rooted in the surveys themselves, which frequently are composed of open-ended questions rather than questions that force respondents to choose one of several specific answers.

Trends in the Data

Clinical Breast Examination/Mammography. The American Cancer Society and the National Cancer Institute recommend that all women have routine clinical breast examinations, although consensus about the precise frequency of the exams has not as yet been reached.

Table 3-13 shows that only about 60 percent of women over age 40 have had a clinical breast exam within the past three years, with no major differences by race/ethnicity. Blacks and Hispanics, however, were over 11 percent more likely than whites never to have had an exam. Women over

TABLE 3-13   Percentage of Women Age 40 and Older Receiving a Clinical Breast Exam, by Race/Ethnicity, 1987

Race	Had Procedure Within Past 3 Years	Had Procedure More Than 3 Years Ago	Had Procedure for Health Problem	Never Had Procedure
All races	58.7	14.6	7.2	19.5
Black (non-Hispanic)	57.9	8.9	5.0	28.2
Hispanic	56.7	11.2	4.0	28.1
White (non-Hispanic)	59.3	15.8	7.8	17.0

SOURCE: Unpublished data from the National Health Interview Survey, National Center for Health Statistics, 1987.

TABLE 3-14   Percentage of Women Age 40 and Older Who Reported
Having Had Mammography, by Race/Ethnicity, 1987

Race	Had Procedure Within Past 3 Years	Had Procedure More Than 3 Years Ago	Had Procedure for Health Problem	Never Had Procedure
All races	23.0	7.3	6.6	63.1
Black (non-Hispanic)	18.1	5.9	5.6	70.3
Hispanic	16.0	7.1	3.1	73.8
White (non-Hispanic)	24.3	7.6	7.0	61.1

SOURCE: Unpublished data from the National Health Interview Survey, National Center
for Health Statistics, 1987.

age 70 are generally less likely to have had an exam, a problem that is more
pronounced for older blacks and Hispanics.   Fifty-one percent of black
women and 47 percent of Hispanic women over the age of 70 have never
had an exam, compared with 29 percent of comparably aged white women
(unpublished data from the NHIS, 1987).

Yet despite age- and race-related differences, the situation has improved
over the past 15 years. The increase was most dramatic for black women
age 60 to 79, whose use of the exam (in the previous two years) jumped 25
percentage points (from 39.1 percent in 1973 to 64.5 percent in 1985). In
all age groups, black women increased their use of breast exams to a greater
extent than white women. By 1985, compared with white women, a larger
percentage of black women were undergoing the screening procedure (Makuc
et al., 1989).

There is general agreement that women over age 50 should receive an
annual mammogram. There is considerable disagreement, however, among
major health organizations about whether regular or any testing should be
done between ages 35 and 49 (U.S. Preventive Services Task Force, 1989;
Hayward et al., 1991a).

The 1987 NHIS data (Tables 3-13 and 3-14) show that fewer than half
as many women had had a mammogram in the past three years as had had a
clinical breast examination. Blacks and Hispanics were less likely to have
had the procedure, and the elderly—especially blacks and Hispanics—were
less likely to have had it than younger women. Seventy-two percent of
white women over age 70 had never had a mammogram—11 percent more
than the comparable figure for younger white women. Among black women
over age 70, 82.4 percent had never had a mammogram. In 1987 slightly
more than 70 percent of all black women age 40 and older had never had a
mammogram. Older Hispanic women were the least likely of any group to

have had a mammogram (86.7 had not). Overall, according to the NHIS data, 73.8 percent of Hispanic women age 40 and over had never had a mammogram.

More recent studies seem to indicate a dramatic increase in mammography screening in all groups, although differences persist by age and race. Mammogram screening increased between 1987 and 1990 (Table 3-15), probably as a result of media coverage and enhanced public health promotion efforts. By 1990, among women over age 40, 64 percent reported having ever had a mammogram, nearly twice the proportion of three years earlier (Centers for Disease Control, 1990).

TABLE 3-15 Percentage of Women Who Reported Ever Having Had a Mammogram, by Race, Age, Income, and Education

Category	MAUS[a] (N = 980)		NKAB[b] (N = 836)		NHIS[c] (N = 6,858)	
	%	95% CI[d]	%	95% CI	%	95% CI
Race						
White	65	62–68	69	65–73	39	38–40
Black	58	47–69	59	52–66	30	28–32
Age (yrs)						
40–49	64	59–69	68	62–74	41	39–43
50–59	71	55–77	70	64–76	44	42–46
60–69	65	59–71	71	65–77	38	36–40
>70	56	49–63	59	51–67	28	27–29
Annual income						
<$25,000	60	55–65	64	59–69	32	31–33
≥$25,000	71	67–76	74	69–79	47	45–49
Education						
Less than high school	58	50–66	58	50–66	25	24–26
High school	65	60–70	67	62–72	41	40–42
Some college	72	66–78	72	66–78	49	47–51
College degree or more	74	68–80	79	72–86	49	47–51
Total	64	61–67	67	64–71	37	36–38

[a]Mammography Attitudes and Usage Study, February 1990; weighted to reflect the age-, education-, and race-specific distribution of U.S. women in 1989.

[b]National Knowledge, Attitudes, and Behavior Survey, April 1989–February 1990; weighted to reflect the age-, education-, and race-specific distribution of U.S. women in 1988.

[c]Unpublished data from the National Health Interview Survey, National Center for Health Statistics, 1987.

[d]Confidence interval.

SOURCE: Centers for Disease Control (1990).

Breast cancer screening varies considerably by region. The 1987 Behavioral Risk Factor Surveillance System, for example, revealed a wide range of mammography usage across the states: from 28.6 percent in New Mexico to 57.5 percent in New Hampshire (Centers for Disease Control, 1989a).

Until recently, with the rise in the number of mammograms, a relatively small proportion of women who had had clinical breast exams went on to have mammograms. For example, data from one large, multisite, survey-based study show that a much higher proportion of women have had a clinical breast exam (between 46 and 76 percent) than have undergone mammography (between 25 and 41 percent; National Cancer Institute, Breast Cancer Screening Consortium, 1990b). Because many women now seem to be self-referring to testing sites, the standard patterns linking clinical exams and mammography may be breaking down, causing some concern about continuity of clinical management.

The DHHS in its Health Objectives for the Year 2000 calls for at least 80 percent of American women age 40 and older to have received a clinical breast exam and a mammogram and 60 percent of women over the age of 50 to have received the two screening tests within the preceding two years (U.S. Public Health Service, 1991). The 1987 baseline rates indicate that only 36 percent of women age 40 and older have ever had both exams and only 25 percent had had both in the previous two years.

The role of economic and noneconomic barriers to screening services needs to be sorted out with further research. In 1985 poor women were 10 to 13 percent less likely than nonpoor women to have undergone a clinical breast exam within the past two years. For most poor women, however, failure to have a clinical breast exam did not appear to be related to a problem of entry into the health care system. For both younger (age 20–39) and older (age 60–79) women, most of the poverty-related differences in the use of screening services occurred among those who had recently visited a health care provider. In fact, data from the NHIS indicate that nearly three-quarters of all women who had not had a breast exam within the past two years reported visiting a physician during that period. Similar results have been obtained from state-based surveys of women's use of health care services (Centers for Disease Control, 1988). These data suggest that even though poor women have contact with the health care system, they may not necessarily receive the services they need, especially screening or preventive services. Whether these data measure poor access to appropriate services or a low quality of care is debatable.

The most frequent reasons for not having a mammogram cited by women in the NHIS were that they had never thought about it or that there was no apparent problem warranting such a procedure. Lack of a recommendation for a mammogram by a physician was the second most frequently cited

TABLE 3-16 Percentage of Women Age 18 and Older Who Reported
Having Had a Pap Smear, by Race/Ethnicity, 1987

Race	Had Procedure Within Past 3 Years	Had Procedure More Than 3 Years Ago	Had Procedure for Health Problem	Never Had Procedure
All races	65.0	15.8	7.8	11.3
Black (non-Hispanic)	68.2	9.2	10.6	11.9
Hispanic	57.7	10.3	7.4	24.7
White (non-Hispanic)	65.7	17.7	7.6	9.0

SOURCE: Unpublished data from the National Health Interview Survey, National Center
for Health Statistics, 1987.

reason (National Cancer Institute, Breast Cancer Screening Consortium, 1990b).
It is not clear how women would have assessed the relative roles of insurance coverage or inability to pay as barriers to access to care because these
questions were not specifically asked.

Pap Tests. In the United States the recommended frequency of Pap
screening for women over age 18 is every one to three years, according to
the discretion of the physician (U.S. Preventive Services Task Force, 1989).
As of 1987 about two-thirds of U.S. women over the age of 18 had had a
Pap smear in the previous three years (Table 3-16). Hispanic women in
general had lower rates of testing, and, as was true for breast cancer screening, women over age 70, particularly black and Hispanic women, were
much less likely than white women to have ever had a Pap test or to have
had one within the past three years. Elderly white women were more than
twice as likely as younger white women never to have had the procedure
(22.6 percent had not had the test). About twice this proportion of same-
age minority women, 43 percent, reported never having had a Pap smear
(analysis of unpublished data from the NHIS, 1987).

Historical trend data on the use of Pap tests are similar to those for the
use of clinical breast exams and mammography. From 1973 to 1985 there
was a small increase (from 63.8 percent in 1973 to 64.8 percent in 1985)
among all women in the use of the test for screening and diagnostic purposes.
For black women, use of the test increased 10 percent (Makuc et al., 1989).

One study that analyzed the 1987 NHIS screening data found that 15.1
percent of Hispanic women had never heard of a Pap test, compared with
4.1 percent of black women and 2.1 percent of white women. Similar,
though less dramatic, differences were observed in the proportion of women
who had undergone the screening procedure. The reason for the gap be-

tween Hispanics and other racial and ethnic groups is unclear, although the authors of the report suggest that cultural avoidance of medical tests by native-Spanish-speakers may be a factor (Harlan et al., 1991). The fault may also lie in a health care delivery system that does not respond appropriately to the health education needs of ethnic communities.

The national health objectives for the year 2000 set a target of increasing to 95 percent the proportion of women 18 and older who have received at least one Pap test. By the year 2000, 80 percent of Hispanic and low-income women should have received a Pap smear within the preceding three years, according to the objectives. The target for women with less than a high school education is 75 percent; for women over age 70, the goal is 70 percent (U.S. Public Health Service, 1991).

As was true for breast cancer screening, data from the NHIS indicate that poor or less educated women are less likely than nonpoor or well-educated women to undergo Pap testing. The majority of reasons cited by women for not obtaining a Pap test reflected a lack of appreciation of the importance of screening rather than cost considerations or lack of access to a physician. A majority (75 percent) of women who had not had the test within the past two years had nevertheless visited a physician during that period. These data raise the question of why the test was not performed during the visit and whether the barrier to screening here is one of poor-quality care rather than access to care.

The usual source of a woman's medical care appears to influence whether she will receive screening for cervical cancer. Women who visited a physician's office were less likely to be screened than those who sought medical care at a health maintenance organization (75.1 percent compared with 85.2 percent, respectively). Only 58.2 percent of women with no regular source of care had had a Pap test within the past three years. Most of the women in this latter group received the test at an outpatient department or public health or community clinic.

A focus-group interview study of physicians found that financial and structural barriers may play an important role in less-than-optimal screening rates. Physicians reported having mixed feelings about pressing poor patients to pay for and undergo screening procedures, particularly if the patients were having difficulty paying their rent. Similarly, when a diabetic patient can barely afford the cost of medication, her physician may be reluctant to urge her to have a mammogram that is expensive and often not covered by insurance. For poor patients, financial problems are exacerbated by the necessity of coping with lack of transportation, child care, and the ability to take time off from work.

An additional aspect that may explain lack of screening is the reluctance of some physicians to perform it, based on their feelings of discomfort or their view that these tests are best left to gynecologists. (Internists and family practitioners, however, are specifically trained in these procedures during residency.) It could be argued that this is not an access problem or that structural deficiencies in the organization of care make it an access problem that reaches beyond the usual financial barriers.

Recommendations

Improved Survey Instruments. The committee believes that surveys about screening services, like the cancer control supplement of the NHIS, should include questions that explore in greater depth the reasons people do not obtain cancer screening services. Survey questions should focus on the effects of insurance coverage and cost issues.

More Frequent Reporting. In those years in which NHIS prevention or cancer supplements are not administered, the Behavioral Risk Factor Surveillance System (BRFSS) should be used to track trends in the data. To accomplish this, questions should be added to the BRFSS surveys to collect information about insurance status, income, and regular source of care.

Outcome Indicator: Incidence of Late-Stage Breast and Cervical Cancers

Late-stage cancers are those that have invaded contiguous tissues and organs or that have spread through the blood or lymphatic system to other parts of the body. Late-stage cancers present a more difficult clinical treatment challenge than those diagnosed at an earlier stage. Late-stage breast and cervical cancers are invariably fatal—therapy in these cases is palliative and not curative.

Discovery of late-stage cancers may indicate the underuse of an effective screening test. Alternatively, or in addition, late-stage cancer may also reflect inappropriate medical follow-up of a diagnosed disease or progression of the cancer in some cases despite appropriate therapy. A recent review article identifies the many steps at which the cervical cancer detection system may fail:

> . . . starting with the initial clinical examination, continuing with the taking of the smear sample and laboratory errors in screening and interpretation, and ending with the clinician's failure to understand the report or take appropriate action and in some instances, with the patient's failure to follow the guidance of the physician. (Koss, 1989)

A large relative difference in late-stage cancer among different groups is an important clue to the existence of problems with access and, potentially, with subsequent treatment. In the case of breast cancer, the diagnosis of late-stage disease may indicate the failure of patients to undergo clinical breast examination or mammography at the recommended intervals. Likewise, the diagnosis of late-stage invasive cervical cancer may indicate underuse of the Pap test.

Measuring the Indicator

Clinically, breast and cervical cancers are grouped into four stages. Ranked in increasing order of severity, they are categorized as in situ, localized, regional, and distant. Diagnoses for any population group of cancers at the last two stages suggest a pattern that may be strongly influenced by barriers and, therefore, a problem in equity of access.

Most national data about cancer incidence come from state and regional tumor registries, which report to the National Cancer Institute's SEER (Surveillance, Epidemiology, and End Results) program. Not all registries report their data to SEER; furthermore, cancer registries in general may not provide a representative sample of the U.S. population. Nonetheless, the SEER system does offer information on more than 1.5 million cases of cancer in geographic areas covering almost 10 percent of the U.S. population. Caution must be exercised, however, in using this data base to generalize about subpopulations. Because the geographic areas included in SEER have changed over the years, data from a consistent set of tumor registries also are reported.

A further shortcoming of the SEER system, for purposes of access monitoring, is that it includes no information about patient income levels or insurance status. Consequently, little is known about these barriers. Income data potentially could be imputed from patient zip code data in tumor registries. Differences in cancer incidence among residents of low- and high-income counties are included in the committee's analysis.

Trends in the Data

Breast Cancer. Breast cancer accounts for 28 percent of all newly diagnosed cancers in women and 18 percent of female cancer deaths (American Cancer Society, 1989). In 1988 the incidence of breast cancer was 112.9 per 100,000 among white women and 96.5 per 100,000 among black women. The age-adjusted death rate from breast cancer for white women was 23 per 100,000; for blacks it was 27 per 100,000. Whites also have higher five-year survival rates than blacks (National Center for Health Statistics, 1990b). These discrepancies are generally attributed to later case finding among blacks. Women who undergo breast cancer screening are about 20 percent more likely than unscreened women to survive five years or longer (U.S. Preventive Services Task Force, 1989).

As Tables 3-17A and 3-17B indicate, a gap has persisted between black

TABLE 3-17A Percentage of Breast Cancers Diagnosed at a Late Stage[a] (total number of staged cases in parentheses) by Period and Race

Period	Whites		Blacks	
All SEER areas				
1973–1977	47.5	(39,978)	56.6	(2,659)
1978–1982	47.4	(46,277)	53.8	(3,511)
1983–1987	39.5	(60,390)	49.8	(4,787)
Selected SEER areas[b]				
1973–1977	48.8	(28,826)	56.8	(2,566)
1978–1982	47.5	(33,783)	53.7	(3,417)
1983–1987	39.2	(44,406)	50.0	(4,644)

SEER, Surveillance, Epidemiology, and End Results (program).

[a]Includes "regional" and "distant." Unstaged cancers are excluded from the denominator.

[b]Atlanta, San Francisco/Oakland, Connecticut, Seattle, and Detroit.

and white women in the proportion of breast cancers diagnosed at late stages. According to SEER program data, the decline in the number of late-stage breast cancers diagnosed among whites in the 1980s has not quite been matched in blacks. Initially, the committee was concerned about time-series analysis that did not include the same group of geographic areas with roughly similar racial compositions over time. However, limiting the analysis to selected tumor registries did not alter the findings.

When high- and low-income areas are compared (Table 3-17B), high-income areas have about 8 percent fewer cases of late-stage cancers in the

TABLE 3-17B Percentage of Breast Cancers Diagnosed at a Late Stage[a] (total number of staged cases in parentheses), by County Per-Capita Income

Period	Low[b]		High[b]	
1973–1977	46.6	(4,270)	46.0	(4,302)
1978–1982	49.2	(4,959)	45.7	(5,116)
1983–1987	43.7	(6,336)	36.1	(6,757)

[a]Includes "regional" and "distant." Unstaged cancers are excluded from the denominator.

[b]Low income is the bottom 10 percent and high income the top 10 percent of all cases grouped by per-capita income of the county of residence.

SOURCE: Unpublished data from the SEER program.

most recent period than in the earliest period. Low-income areas improved only about a third as much after a period of increases in the middle period.

Cervical Cancer. Five thousand women die annually from cervical cancer. The incidence was twice as high among black women (15.8 per 100,000) as it was among white women (7.8 per 100,000) from 1983 through 1987. Mortality was nearly three times as high among blacks during the same period (6.4 per 100,000 for blacks compared with 2.3 per 100,000 for whites). From 1981 through 1986 the five-year survival rate for white women was 67.3 percent; for black women it was 57.1 percent.

Early diagnosis is closely linked to reduced rates of invasive cervical cancer. Such diagnosis can reduce the mortality rate by up to 75 percent (U.S. Public Health Service, 1991). In one study the cumulative incidence of invasive cervical cancer was reduced almost 84 percent when Pap tests were conducted every five years; it was reduced nearly 93 percent when the interval between testing was reduced to two years (International Agency for Research on Cancer, Working Group on Evaluation of Cervical Cancer Screening Programmes, 1986).

Among whites the proportion of cases of late-stage (regional and distant) cervical cancer remained approximately the same in the 1970s and 1980s. In contrast, the proportion of late-stage diagnoses for blacks, which was approximately the same as that for whites in the mid-1970s, nearly doubled by the mid-1980s (Table 3-18A). With respect to income levels, only a small difference persists over time, and that gap appears to be narrowing (Table 3-18B). As Figure 3-2 illustrates, survival is strongly linked to the stage of diagnosis.

TABLE 3-18A Percentage of Cervical Cancers Diagnosed at a Late Stage[a] (total number of staged cases in parentheses), by Period and Race

Period	Whites		Blacks	
All SEER areas				
1973–1977	8.5	(19,594)	8.5	(4,113)
1978–1982	9.4	(19,429)	11.3	(3,681)
1983–1987	8.2	(21,585)	15.0	(3,148)
Selected SEER areas[b]				
1973–1977	8.2	(13,792)	8.3	(4,014)
1978–1982	8.7	(14,312)	11.3	(3,591)
1983–1987	7.8	(15,464)	15.0	(3,050)

SEER, Surveillance, Epidemiology, and End Results (program).

[a]Includes "regional" and "distant." Unstaged cancers are excluded from the denominator.

[b]Atlanta, San Francisco/Oakland, Connecticut, Seattle, and Detroit.

TABLE 3-18B Percentage of Cervical Cancers Diagnosed at a Late Stage[a] (total number of staged cases in parentheses), by County Per-Capita Income

Period	Low[b]		High[b]	
1973–1977	10.3	(2,337)	7.8	(2,139)
1978–1982	10.3	(2,332)	7.2	(2,064)
1983–1987	9.4	(2,627)	8.5	(2,274)

[a]Includes "regional" and "distant." Unstaged cancers are excluded from the denominator.

[b]Low income is the bottom 10 percent and high income the top 20 percent of all cases distributed by per-capita income of the county of residence.

SOURCE: Unpublished data from the SEER program.

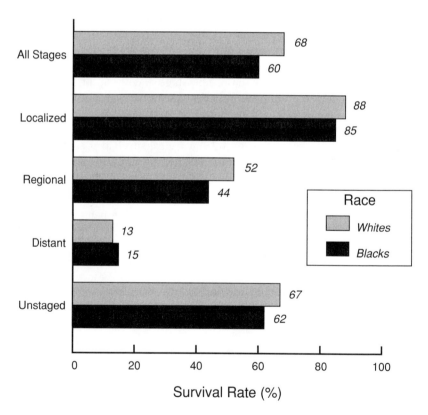

FIGURE 3-2 Five-year survival rates by stage for cancer of the cervix uteri, 1981–1986. SOURCE: National Cancer Institute (1990a).

Recommendations

Enhancing the SEER Data. The SEER data should contain more background information, including the socioeconomic and insurance status of patients. In the interim, zip code analyses to impute income must suffice.

A Clearinghouse for Analyzing Access Problems. The committee believes that the nation needs a clearinghouse of cancer registry data that can be used to analyze access problems. It is beyond the scope of this committee's charge to determine whether this could or should be achieved through expansion of the SEER program or whether some other organizational structure or cooperative arrangement would be better suited to accomplish this objective.

Research Studies. More detailed studies are needed to determine why increases in the use of screening tests by blacks are not reflected in improvements in stage of diagnosis, mortality, and survival.

OBJECTIVE 4: REDUCING THE EFFECTS OF CHRONIC DISEASES AND PROLONGING LIFE

Utilization Indicator: Continuing Care for Chronic Diseases

Many of the reasons people use medical care are related to the treatment of chronic conditions. These diseases are usually not self-limiting and are ongoing over an extended period. Chronic diseases often limit how well a person functions in society. Many chronic diseases include episodes of acute illness followed by quiescent periods.

Diabetes, asthma, congestive heart disease, and hypertension are examples of chronic diseases that, without regular medical management (follow-up care), can result in repeated hospitalization, premature disability, and death. Adverse consequences of chronic conditions can occur with or without regular medical care, but negative consequences are more common when regular care is absent. Even when life cannot be extended, health care can contribute to improved functioning and can minimize discomfort.

Continuing care for a chronic illness may include periodic tests to monitor a patient's health status, nutritional and other types of counseling to reduce or eliminate patient behaviors that may be harmful to health, and necessary medications and medical and surgical procedures. Underuse of the health care system by those with chronic diseases—as reflected by few or irregular physician visits or a less than optimal regimen of care—may indicate an access problem.

Diabetes offers a useful illustration of how a utilization measure (follow-up care) may be applied to a chronic disease condition. Diabetes is a relatively common illness. Some 7 million people in the United States have been diagnosed with the disease; another 5 million may have it without knowing it (U.S. Public Health Service, 1991). Although few people die from diabetes directly, the disease is a major indirect contributor to mortality in the United States. In 1987 diabetes was the sixth leading underlying cause of death from disease (National Center for Health Statistics, 1987). Two of the most common diabetes-related causes of death are cardiovascular disease (accounting for somewhat more than half of all deaths) and diabetic ketoacidosis.

Standard treatment for diabetes includes diet, exercise, and the administration of insulin or oral hypoglycemic agents. Physicians prescribe one or a mix of these three treatment modalities, depending on the severity of illness and other patient factors (Drury et al., 1981).

Good health practices, such as not smoking and drinking alcohol only in moderation, and the use of preventive health services, such as regular eye and dental exams, stress management of blood pressure, and control of lipid problems, also are important for maintaining the health of the diabetic patient. In addition, because most care for diabetes rests with the individual patient, patient and family knowledge about the disease and compliance with a recommended course of treatment are crucial.

Thus, continuing contact with a regular health care provider is essential for the effective control of diabetes. A breakdown in patient management can have a significant adverse impact on the speed and severity of the disease's effects on a patient's health status. Similar examples can be cited for other chronic illnesses for which regular medical care can have beneficial results.

Measuring the Indicator

There is no direct, routinely available way to measure the use of particular follow-up health care services for specific chronic diseases, like diabetes, that could be used to measure barriers to access. Periodically, however, the extent to which patients with a particular disease have contact with the personal health care system has been documented through supplements to the NHIS. NHIS supplemental data collection on diabetes was performed in 1976 and 1989. The 1989 NHIS also included supplements on mental health services and digestive disorders. However, data from the 1989 supplements were not available in time to analyze them for this report.

Disease-specific surveys with appropriate questions on barriers are the preferred approach for precise monitoring of access problems. Absent such studies, it is possible nonetheless to make inferences about the adequacy of follow-up care for chronic diseases in general. The NHIS can be used to measure physician contacts with persons who judge themselves to be in fair to poor health as opposed to excellent, very good, and good health. People who rate their health status as fair or poor often are afflicted with serious chronic health conditions that can be helped by medical management. Perceived health status may be the best indirect variable for measuring chronic, serious, yet manageable conditions like diabetes (Pope, 1988). The committee's analysis of the NHIS indicates that nonelderly people who are in fair to poor health, compared with those in good to excellent health, are two-and-a-half times as likely to be unable to carry out major activities of living. They also report four times the number of chronic conditions.

The committee used two measures of physician use in its analysis of chronic illness care. The first was a stringent measure of access to care that focused on entry into the system—that is, whether an individual had had any contact with a physician in the past year. Respondents to the health interview survey were asked to report the interval since the last time they had a physician contact in person or by telephone. The second measure focused on the comparative frequency of use, namely, the average number of contacts per year by insurance status, income level, and other characteristics relevant to access.

Trends in the Data

Having health care coverage makes a major difference in whether persons who rate their health as fair or poor have at least one physician contact within a year. Table 3-19 compares such people with different types of insurance coverage. In 1989 the uninsured were more than twice as likely as those with private health insurance, Medicaid, or Medicare to go without physician contact. Those with both Medicare coverage and supplemental private insurance were even more likely to have had contact with a doctor. In general, there was only a very slight increase in access to physicians for all coverage groups during the 1980s.

For the uninsured in fair to poor health, level of income can be a major factor in determining physician contact (see Table 3-20). The uninsured at the lowest income level are more than twice as likely as those with middle-range incomes not to have had a physician contact in the past year. For most of those with coverage, level of income is only marginally related to physician use, with one exception: Medicare recipients without private insurance are much less likely to contact a physician if they have a low income.

Once insurance and income are taken into account, other potential barriers to access do not seem to have a consistent effect on who contacts a physician. Differences in the proportions of those without a physician contact according to race, ethnicity, and geographic location generally disappear when income and insurance are taken into account. One exception is

TABLE 3-19   Percentage of People in Poor/Fair Health Who Did Not Contact a Physician in the Past Year, by Health Care Coverage, Selected Years

Insurance Coverage[a]	1980	1986	1989
Uninsured	24	25	22
Private health insurance	12	11	9
Medicaid only	11	6	8
Medicare only	14	11	10
Medicare and private health insurance	9	6	5
All others	13	7	8

[a]Insurance definitions are as follows: Medicaid only—if the person has a current Medicaid card or is covered by Aid to Families with Dependent Children, Supplemental Security Income, or public assistance and has no other insurance coverage; Medicare plus other health insurance—Medicare plus either private insurance, Medicaid, or CHAMPUS/ Veterans Administration or military health insurance. Private health insurance includes only people who reported private insurance and no other types of insurance.

SOURCE: Unpublished data from the National Health Interview Survey, National Center for Health Statistics, 1980, 1986, 1989.

TABLE 3-20   Percentage of People in Poor/Fair Health Who Did Not Contact a Physician in the Past Year, by Type of Insurance and Income Level, 1989

Insurance Coverage[a]	Lowest Income	Lower- Middle Income	Middle Income	Highest Income
Uninsured	28	19	12	*
Private health insurance	12	11	8	8
Medicaid only	10	7	*	*
Medicare only	18	12	8	*
Medicare and private health insurance	6	6	5	5

[a]Insurance definitions are as follows: Medicaid only—if the person has a current Medicaid card or is covered by Aid to Families with Dependent Children, Supplemental Security Income, or public assistance and has no other insurance coverage; Medicare plus other health insurance—Medicare plus either private insurance, Medicaid, or CHAMPUS/ Veterans Administration or military health insurance. Private health insurance includes only people who reported private insurance and no other types of insurance.

*Estimates for which the relative standard error exceeds 30 percent are not reported.

SOURCE: Unpublished data from the National Health Interview Survey, National Center for Health Statistics, 1989.

rural residents who are both uninsured and at the lowest income level; this is the group that is least likely to have had a physician contact. Thirty-five percent of rural residents had not had a contact, compared with 24 percent of those who lived in similar circumstance but in a metropolitan area.

As Table 3-21 shows, lack of insurance as a barrier is somewhat muted for sick children under age 5. Children over age 5 without insurance, however, are more than twice as likely to have had no physician contact, despite how their health is perceived, than older children who have insurance.

Among persons who rated themselves as being in poor or fair health in 1989 (the committee's indirect indicator of underlying chronic disease), the average number of physician visits per year (estimated from a two-week recall question) by those with private health care coverage (14.8) or Medicaid (16.9) was substantially higher than the number of visits by people without insurance (9.1; Table 3-22). For persons with Medicaid or private health insurance, blacks reported fewer visits than whites with the same health status.

Although a stepwise relationship can be found between physician contacts and income levels, for the most part this relationship is not very strong when health care insurance coverage status is taken into account (Table 3-23). The difference between the high- and low-income categories for the privately insured indicates the probable effect of coinsurance and deductibles. One possible explanation of the high utilization of physician services by Medicaid recipients in the lower middle income group is the likelihood that they have high-cost illnesses that qualify them for the program.

TABLE 3-21 Percentage of People in Poor/Fair Health Who Have Not Contacted a Physician in the Past Year, by Age and Health Care Coverage, 1989

Age	Uninsured	Medicaid Only	Private Health Insurance
0–4	6	1	3
5–17	17	10	8
18–44	24	10	11
45–64	20	6	9

Insurance definitions are as follows: Medicaid only—if the person has a current Medicaid card or is covered by Aid to Families with Dependent Children, Supplemental Security Income, or public assistance and has no other insurance coverage; Medicare plus other health insurance—Medicare plus either private insurance, Medicaid, or CHAMPUS/Veterans Administration or military health insurance. Private health insurance includes only people who reported private insurance and no other types of insurance.

SOURCE: Unpublished data from the National Health Interview Survey, National Center for Health Statistics, 1989.

TABLE 3-22   Average Number of Annual Physician Contacts by Those Who Report Fair/Poor Health, by Health Care Coverage and Race/Ethnicity, 1989

Insurance Coverage[a]	Total	White	Black	Hispanic	Non-Hispanic
Uninsured	9.1	9.6	7.8	9.7	6.0
Private health insurance	14.8	15.6	12.0	15.2	10.7
Medicaid only	16.9	20.8	11.4	17.5	14.4
Medicare	12.9	12.8	12.7	12.7	*
Medicare and private health insurance	16.5	15.9	20.0	16.2	*

[a]Insurance definitions are as follows: Medicaid only—if the person has a current Medicaid card or is covered by Aid to Families with Dependent Children, Supplemental Security Income, or public assistance and has no other insurance coverage; Medicare plus other health insurance—Medicare plus either private insurance, Medicaid, or CHAMPUS/Veterans Administration or military health insurance. Private health insurance includes only people who reported private insurance and no other types of insurance.

*Estimates for which the relative standard error exceeds 30 percent are not reported.

SOURCE: Unpublished data from the National Health Interview Survey, National Center for Health Statistics, 1989.

Recommendations

Longitudinal Survey of Individuals with Chronic Diseases. Longitudinal surveys are the most effective way to monitor the effect of access barriers on the ability of chronic disease sufferers to obtain necessary and appropriate care. The epidemiological follow-up studies of the National Health and Nutrition Examination Survey should be explored for their potential to serve this purpose. Several advantages of this approach are detailed below.

• First, it would be useful to track diseases that are highly prevalent among groups that are likely to face barriers to access. Using the example of diabetes, the Secretary's Task Force on Black and Minority Health noted that "diabetes exemplifies the difference in health status between whites and minority groups. . . . Blacks, native Americans, Hispanic Americans, and Asian Americans suffer a disproportionate share of the disease, its effects, and the complications that arise from it" (U.S. Department of Health and Human Services, 1986). The task force report identifies demonstration programs that have decreased the adverse consequences of the dis-

TABLE 3-23 Average Number of Physician Contacts by Those Who Report Fair/Poor Health, by Family Income and Health Care Coverage, 1989

Insurance Coverage[b]	Levels of Family Income[a]			
	Bottom	Lower Middle	Middle	Upper
Uninsured	7.1	11.5	7.8	*
Private health insurance	13.2	13.4	16.5	19.0
Medicaid only	14.7	21.4	*	*
Medicare only	14.0	13.7	16.9	*
Medicare plus other insurance	18.1	16.1	15.5	21.8
Total	13.5	14.7	15.8	19.3

[a]Income groupings are based on family income and are defined separately for people under 65 and for those 65 and older. For those under 65, bottom is less than $9,000 (10.5%), lower middle is $9,000–$24,999 (29.2%), middle is $25,000–$49,999 (39.3%), and upper is $50,000 or more (21.0%). For the elderly, the corresponding figures are bottom, less than $6,000 (9.6%); lower middle, $6,000–$15,999 (51.5%); middle, $16,000–$34,999 (27.3%); and upper, $35,000 or more (11.6%).

[b]Insurance definitions are as follows: Medicaid only—if the person has a current Medicaid card or is covered by Aid to Families with Dependent Children, Supplemental Security Income, or public assistance and has no other insurance coverage; Medicare plus other health insurance—Medicare plus either private insurance, Medicaid, or CHAMPUS/Veterans Administration or military health insurance. Private health insurance includes only people who reported private insurance and no other types of insurance.

*Estimates for which the relative standard error exceeds 30 percent are not reported.

SOURCE: Unpublished data from the National Health Interview Survey, National Center for Health Statistics, 1989.

ease by providing patients with continuing and meaningful contact with the personal health care system.

• Second, by comparing population groups with the same disease, it is easier to control for severity and changing treatment patterns that may confound analyses of service use.

• Third, the use of specific services that make a difference for health outcomes can be tracked. For example, diabetics should have their blood pressure and blood serum lipids monitored routinely, and they should visit an ophthalmologist to be checked for proliferative retinopathy.

The committee recommends that the federal government or a foundation support a longitudinal survey of the type described.

Modifications of the NHIS. The lead time for a new national survey can be extensive. In the interim the committee recommends that the regular series of the NHIS be modified to include access-related questions about specific diseases. Among other areas, the questions should address the types of follow-up care known to have a positive effect on prognosis.

The National Center for Health Statistics should determine whether this modification could best be done through changes in core sections of the survey (e.g., supplementary questions to the condition list) or through regularly rotating supplements that include appropriate access questions. The anticipated redesign of the NHIS core will be an opportunity to consider these options.

Utilization Indicator: Use of High-Cost Discretionary Care

For many medical and surgical procedures, there is general agreement in the medical community about the clinical criteria that guide their use. For other procedures, however, physicians may have legitimate disagreements about their appropriate utilization. These latter procedures are termed referral sensitive because their performance depends on the judgment of the physicians who provide first-contact care and who may or may not decide to refer a patient elsewhere for more specialized treatment. Whether a procedure is indeed performed also depends on the judgment of the surgeon or specialist to whom the patient is referred. The extent to which these referral decisions are influenced, directly or indirectly, by the patient's insurance status, race, or social class may reflect a problem with equity of access.

Some referral-sensitive surgeries, like organ transplantation, can affect patient survival. Other procedures, like hip transplants or breast reconstructions, may improve physical or social functioning without necessarily extending the patient's life span. Although people do not die of osteoarthritis of the hip, the burden of pain and suffering is extremely high. Total hip replacement is not discretionary in the sense of relieving pain and suffering, but it may be treated as such by the medical care system in some cases.

For most of its work, the committee has selected indicators that are agreed to be effective and generally applicable to easily identifiable groups such as women of certain ages or children. In contrast, referral-sensitive procedures constitute a wide area of medical practice in which judgments about effectiveness or appropriateness are difficult to make without a detailed case-by-case review. Yet growing pressure to eliminate ineffective or inappropriate procedures in the name of cost and quality control is working to ensure that these judgments are, indeed, made. An access monitoring tool must be able to measure how these judgments are affecting differential use of discretionary procedures among subpopulations.

As an indicator, referral-sensitive surgeries reach beyond a person's entry into the personal health care system to assess a second level of access—expensive discretionary procedures. That this is a problem worth monitoring emerges from the medical literature, which contains examples of medical and surgical procedures for which there are differences in utilization according to patient health insurance status, race, and other sociodemographic factors.

One national study of hospital discharge abstracts revealed that uninsured patients were between 29 and 75 percent less likely than those with insurance to undergo one of five high-cost or high-discretion procedures: coronary artery bypass surgery, total knee replacement, total hip replacement, stapedectomy, and surgical correction of strabismus (Hadley et al., 1991). Similar findings were reported for the use of angiography, angioplasty, and cardiac bypass grafting among patients treated in Massachusetts hospitals. Low-income patients, the uninsured, and blacks had lower rates of use than their more wealthy, insured white counterparts for all three procedures (Wenneker et al., 1990). In Maryland it was shown that population rates for discretionary orthopedic, vascular, and laryngologic surgery increased with income. Coronary and carotid artery surgery rates were two to three times higher for whites than blacks (Gittelsohn et al., 1991).

Lung cancer treatment also has been shown to vary according to insurance status, both for those who undergo surgical treatment and those who are treated instead with radiation, chemotherapy, or both. Greenberg and colleagues (1988) showed that in both groups those with private insurance were about 50 percent more likely to receive treatment than those without insurance. They also noted that nonclinical factors, such as insurance, may be particularly important in guiding physician choice of treatment in diseases like lung cancer in which the benefit of any therapy is minimal. Surgery and radiation therapy both entail long hospital stays and considerable expense, factors that may discourage their use in patients who lack insurance (Greenberg et al., 1988).

An IOM study of Medicare's end-stage renal disease program documented access problems inherent even in a "near-universal" entitlement program (Institute of Medicine, 1991). Those ineligible for benefits were found to be disproportionately poor and minority. Various features of the program's organization and payment policies created barriers to access for many patients. One of these barriers is particularly relevant in this discussion because it illustrates the difficulty of interpreting differences in access to referral-sensitive procedures. In a study of dialysis patients and their information-seeking behavior, black patients were at a particular disadvantage in obtaining transplantation. They felt less competent than whites to decide about the procedure, were less inclined to discuss the matter with their nephrologist, and seldom had access to a transplant surgeon. If a fuller understanding of access barriers is to be gained, more in-depth analysis of the reasons for differential use, especially of discretionary procedures, is needed.

Measuring the Indicator

The committee chose to base its measurement of access to referral-sensitive surgeries on differences in the rates at which these procedures are performed among various subpopulations. The major focus of analysis is the differences among populations of high- and low-income neighborhoods in 11 states (see Table 3-24). The potential effects of race and insurance status on the likelihood of receiving these procedures also are considered.

The committee collaborated in this analysis with the United Hospital Fund Ambulatory Care Access Project (ACAP) and the Codman Research Group. Together, these groups selected a set of five procedures for analysis: hip/joint replacement, breast reconstruction after mastectomy, pacemaker insertion, coronary artery bypass surgery, and coronary angioplasty.

As with many access monitoring indicators, the major methodological issues in the use of referral-sensitive procedures involve the need to control for alternative explanations of differences in utilization rates by income,

TABLE 3-24 Referral-Sensitive Surgeries for Selected Conditions, by Zip Code/Income Groups, 1988, 11 States[a]

Condition	Low-Income Admissions/ 1,000 Population	High-Income Admissions/ 1,000 Population	Ratio, Low/High
Hip/joint replacement	0.26	0.29	0.90
Breast reconstruction after mastectomy	0.02	0.10	0.20
Pacemaker insertion	0.22	0.23	0.96
Coronary artery bypass surgery	0.26	0.44	0.59
Coronary angioplasty	0.22	0.51	0.43
Total referrals	0.98	1.57	0.62

[a]California, Florida, Illinois, Massachusetts, Nevada, New Hampshire, New Jersey, New York, Oregon, Vermont, Washington.

SOURCE: Joint data and analysis by the Codman Research Group, the Ambulatory Care Access Project (United Hospital Fund of New York), and the IOM Access Monitoring Committee.

race, and insurance status. As noted previously, these differences may be due not to access barriers but to levels of severity of disease, or of prevalence, patients' social environment, and compliance. Moreover, in view of the discretionary nature of these procedures, patients may forgo the surgery option not because of cost but because of concerns about risks and potential discomfort. The extent to which patient preferences and risk aversion are related to their use of these procedures is not well understood.

Differences in the utilization of certain surgical procedures according to race, income, and other factors have been well documented. What is not clear is what proportion of the differences may be due to overutilization of such procedures by those in the more "favored" groups—whites and those with health insurance, for example.

Research on appropriateness of use suggests that one-quarter to one-third of all medical procedures may be of little or no benefit to patients (Brook and Lohr, 1986). Many third-party payers have instituted utilization management strategies to reduce outlays for inappropriate health care services. Still, because utilization management is in its infancy, there are many procedures for which information about appropriateness is unavailable. The challenge will be to determine whether inappropriate use explains why some groups appear to be underutilizing certain procedures relative to other groups.

Trends in the Data

Because the methodology for this utilization indicator is new, there are no year-to-year trend data. Table 3-24 presents aggregated data for 1988 from the states in the committee's sample of hospital discharge data bases. The ratios in the table represent a comparison of low-income (60 percent or more of the population with incomes below $15,000) and high-income (10 percent or less of the incomes below $15,000) zip codes. A ratio of 1.0 indicates no difference between the two income groups; ratios of less than 1.0 signify that individuals from high-income areas undergo the procedures at a higher rate than those from low-income areas.

The summary figure of 0.62 suggests that, when all the referral-sensitive procedures are combined, people from poor areas appear to be less likely to obtain these services than people from more affluent areas. The most marked differences found were for breast reconstruction (0.20), coronary artery bypass grafts (0.59), and coronary angiography (0.43). The data did not reveal major differences for hip/joint replacement and pacemaker insertion.

The relative rates of admission for referral-sensitive procedures are also comparatively low for zip code areas composed predominantly of black residents, even in those areas with higher-than-average incomes. This confirms research demonstrating a lower rate of use of cardiac procedures among blacks with private insurance or Medicare compared with whites who are similarly insured (Wenneker and Epstein, 1989). White Medicare recipients are three times more likely than black Medicare recipients to receive coronary artery bypass graft surgery and angioplasty. White Medicare recipients are also more likely than blacks to have magnetic resonance imaging (MRI) scans rather than the less costly computed tomography (CT) scans (Boutwell and Mitchell, 1991).

Recommendations

Standards for Appropriate Use. Increasing attention is being paid to outcomes research and the development of clinical practice guidelines. As techniques become established for determining the appropriateness of use of certain medical procedures, interpreting differences in use among subpopulations will become easier. For example, these techniques will allow us to distinguish problems in access from overutilization of services by specific populations.

Improved Data Availability. Researchers who are seeking improvements in clinical data bases for use in outcomes research should work with those interested in access research to determine whether there are mutually beneficial opportunities for enhancing these data bases. An issue of interest to both groups, for instance, might be the addition of information to the discharge abstract, which would help to measure severity more accurately.

Outcome Indicator: Avoidable Hospitalization for Chronic Diseases

For the purposes of this indicator, "avoidable hospitalizations" are those that might not have occurred had the patient received effective, timely, and continuous outpatient (ambulatory) medical care for certain chronic disease conditions. Although hospital admission rates are generally a utilization measure, they are used here as a proxy for health conditions that have deteriorated to the point where hospitalization is required.

Ongoing medical management can effectively control the severity and progression of a number of chronic diseases, even if the diseases themselves cannot be prevented. An advanced stage of a chronic disease that requires hospitalization may indicate the existence of one or more barriers to access to the personal health care system. Thus, hospital admissions for certain conditions are a potentially useful indicator of the performance of the ambulatory health care system. High rates of admissions for conditions related to treatable chronic diseases in particular may provide indirect evidence of serious patient access problems or deficiencies in outpatient management.

Measuring the Indicator

In the indicator for use of discretionary procedures (discussed above), the committee used hospital discharge data to identify income differences in the utilization of referral-sensitive procedures. The same technique can be used to create an outcome indicator for utilization of ambulatory care. In this case, hospital admission represents a failure in outpatient management rather than use of a service. By comparing different income groups by zip code, one can roughly compare the relative frequency of outpatient management failures by income status.

The committee has identified a specific set of diagnoses representing conditions that, with timely and effective outpatient care, normally would not result in a hospital admission. No matter how timely or effective outpatient medical management may be, a certain amount of hospitalization among patients with chronic diseases is expected. If differences in disease prevalence are taken into account, however, there should be no major differences in hospital admission rates according to income level, insurance status, or race.

Accurate diagnostic data may be obtained by using the disease coding system of the ninth edition of the *International Classification of Diseases* (ICD-9; U.S. Department of Health and Human Services, 1991), which provides detailed diagnosis information. The aim is to identify diagnoses that are clearly related to the need to treat a patient in the hospital. Furthermore, ICD-9 codes allow fairly precise selection of conditions that are likely to be related to the adequacy of outpatient management.

The source of diagnostic data is the hospital discharge summary. These summaries, at a minimum, provide up to five diagnostic codes (for patients with multiple diagnoses); three procedure codes; and the patient's age, sex, and race. Currently, about two dozen states have centralized hospital discharge data bases, which allows comparisons to be made among all hospitals in a state. Eleven were selected for the committee's analysis.[2]

Discharge summaries also report a patient's zip code and the expected source of payment. Zip code information permits the matching of diagnosis and procedure with the demographics of the patient's neighborhood, allowing a rough estimate of personal income. Thus, the measure of the avoidable hospitalization indicator is a population-based rate using zip codes grouped by income to approximate differences in the variables of interest (income, insurance, and race). To account for differences among population groupings, the data are adjusted for age and sex. The committee focused initially on admissions for those under age 65, because most of the elderly have Medicare coverage.

---

[2] The states selected are California, Florida, Illinois, Massachusetts, Nevada, New Hampshire, New Jersey, New York, Oregon, Vermont, and Washington.

As noted in the discussion of the previous indicator, the committee collaborated with the Ambulatory Care Access Project of the United Hospital Fund of New York in selecting a set of chronic-disease-related diagnoses that are potentially sensitive to outpatient care across a range of clinical areas and patient-age cohorts. Appendix D contains a list of those conditions. The Codman Research Group provided hospital discharge data in a form that was suitable for analysis.

Information about household income generally is not collected when a patient enters the hospital. Income can be estimated by matching patient zip codes, which are recorded on hospital discharge summaries, with zip-code-area income-level information available from the Census Bureau. The problem with this indirect approach of measuring patient income is that it is imprecise. Small pockets of the poor in otherwise high-income areas, as well as dispersal of the poor across a wide region, can be particularly problematic.

Although information about health insurance status is included on the standard hospital discharge form, there are no good data on insurance status by geographic area. Without such "denominator" data, it is difficult to know whether hospital admission rates for ambulatory-sensitive conditions are higher than expected, given the levels of insurance in an area. Recent work by Wenneker and colleagues (1990), however, seems to indicate that comparisons by insurance coverage status provide results similar to those of the income analysis, which is probably due to correlation of the two barriers.

Finally, few data are available that shed any light on the relative importance of a variety of factors that appear to contribute to delayed or inadequate outpatient care. One such factor, the criteria used by physicians to admit patients to the hospital, has been examined by the ACAP. It might be expected that many physicians would have a lower threshold for admitting low-income patients than for high-income patients. This might be the case either because of differences in the level of clinical training for physicians in poorer areas or because of physician concerns about lack of access by poor patients to regular outpatient services, their weak family support systems, or their sometimes less-than-optimal compliance with recommended outpatient treatment. However, the ACAP data for New York City indicate that differences in patient severity are unlikely to account for the differences in admission rates seen between low-income and high-income areas (Billings et al., 1991).

Trends in the Data

Table 3-25 lists the discharge diagnoses for the chronic conditions chosen for the analysis, the admission rates (per 1,000 population) for low- and high-income zip codes, and a comparison of those rates in the form of a

TABLE 3-25 Admission Rates for Selected Ambulatory-Care-Sensitive Conditions, by Zip Code/Income Groups, 1988, 11 States[a]

Condition	Low-Income Admissions/ 1,000 Population	High-Income Admissions/ 1,000 Population	Ratio, Low/High Income
Angina	1.71	0.63	2.71
Asthma	5.44	0.94	5.79
Grand mal status	0.74	0.20	3.70
Chronic obstructive pulmonary disease	0.73	0.20	3.65
Congestive heart failure	2.13	0.35	6.09
Convulsions	1.17	0.30	3.90
Diabetes DKA/hyperosmolar coma	0.78	0.19	4.11
With complications	1.34	0.28	4.79
Without complications	0.08	0.02	4.00
Hypoglycemia	0.14	0.03	4.67
Hypertension	0.84	0.11	7.64
Total	15.10	3.25	4.65

[a]California, Florida, Illinois, Massachusetts, Nevada, New Hampshire, New Jersey, New York, Oregon, Vermont, Washington.

SOURCE: Joint data and analysis by the Codman Research Group, the Ambulatory Care Access Project (United Hospital Fund of New York), and the IOM Access Monitoring Committee.

ratio. All of the ambulatory-care-sensitive admission rates were substantially higher for low-income areas. The greatest differences—ranging in size from six- to sevenfold—were related to admissions for congestive heart failure, hypertension, and asthma. However, even angina, the diagnosis with the lowest ratio (and thus the least difference between rates), showed income differences of almost threefold. The overall average rate of difference was 4.65.

Billings and his colleagues (1991), examining New York City discharge data, looked at the effects of race, substance abuse, and prevalence of disease conditions on the differences between high- and low-income areas. They found that predominantly black middle-income zip codes resembled other middle-class areas but that poor black areas had consistently higher admission rates than comparable white low-income zip codes. By examining secondary diagnoses of alcohol and drug dependence/abuse, they noted that, although alcohol/substance abuse explains some of the differentials for the 22- to 44-year-old population with respect to bacterial pneumonia and tuberculosis, for the most part such abuse has little impact on rates for most of the conditions chosen for this analysis. Finally, in terms of differences in disease prevalence, the research group looked at asthma and diabetes—two conditions for which data on prevalence are available through the NHIS. Depending on the age group, differences in prevalence between high- and low-income populations ranged from 1.35 to 2.36 times higher for low-income age cohorts with asthma and from 1.15 to 2.96 times higher for low-income cohorts with diabetes. Prevalence thus explains only a portion of the four- to fivefold differences between income groupings for these two conditions.

Recommendations

Hospital Discharge Data Systems. States that do not have centralized hospital discharge data bases should develop them. In addition to their value for the types of analyses suggested by this committee, the data bases will be useful for future research on costs and quality of care.

Expanding Data Elements in the Discharge Abstract. As recommended previously, states should consider the feasibility of adding additional elements to the discharge abstract, especially information to measure the severity of illness and income.

Further Research. The committee believes that more detailed studies of patients and admitting physicians are needed to sort out the relative contribution of the various factors, including access to primary care, that lead to hospitalization for chronic disease-related conditions. Items of particular interest include the timeliness and quality of outpatient care, patient characteristics, and physician admitting practices. Studies focusing on better measurement of continuity of care and the effect of site of care (walk-in clinics, physician's offices, hospital clinics, community health centers, emergency departments) also should be considered.

Outcome Indicator: Access-Related Excess Mortality

The access-related excess mortality rate is the number of deaths per 100,000 population that are thought to be the result of access problems. The estimate is based on a comparison of two groups in the population—one that is believed to have relatively good access and one that is considered likely to experience barriers to access. Because data are available (Stoto, 1992), the population groups of particular focus for this measure are blacks and whites.

It has been well documented that, compared with whites, blacks in the United States have a disproportionately high mortality rate from chronic disease. Some of the difference may be the result of increased levels of behavioral risk factors among blacks, such as higher rates of smoking (U.S. Public Health Service, 1991). Physiological factors, such as a genetic predisposition to high blood pressure, may also play a role. Problems known to have an effect on access to health care, such as lack of insurance, poverty, and low educational attainment, may be important as well.

If the effects on black mortality of physiological and behavioral risk factors can be statistically "removed," the remaining difference in the death rate between blacks and whites (for diseases that can be managed with medical care) may be attributable, in large part, to differences in access to health care. The statistical calculations necessary to control for the effects of these factors require a number of assumptions that can be questioned. The methodological challenges that must be overcome to enhance the utility of this indicator are discussed below and in the recommendations section. In addition to questions of methodology, some conceptual issues also need to be resolved. Foremost among these is the dilemma of how to handle chronic disease behavioral risk factors—for example, hypertension—that could be ameliorated by treatment or care and whose presence may indicate barriers to access to health care services. Yet despite such conceptual and technical issues, the committee believes that the approach presented here, albeit on a developmental basis, will be an improvement over the unadjusted comparisons of death rates that are frequently cited.

Measuring the Indicator

A critical component in calculating an access-related mortality rate is the adjustment for risk factors. If access were the only factor that distinguished black and white mortality, there would be no need to adjust for risk factors. For example, one would not compare the mortality rates at two hospitals without first adjusting for the relative risks of death for each patient, including age, severity of illness, and procedures undergone. Similarly, one cannot compare how the personal health care system (the hospital in the above analogy) performs for blacks compared with whites (one hospital's patients compared with another's) without first taking into account the differences (in terms of behavior, physiology, and environmental surroundings) between blacks and whites.

Fortunately, the results of epidemiological follow-up studies of health examination surveys performed in the 1970s provide a basis for measuring how six major risk factors interact and affect mortality for the two races. Applying these results to the black mortality rate reveals the level of mortality that blacks would experience if the pattern of their risk factors was the same as that for whites.

In sum, access-related excess mortality is calculated by subtracting two rates. The rate is the actual rate of death in the group with higher mortality (in this case blacks). The second lower rate is an estimate of what the black death rate would be if blacks had the same pattern of risk factors as whites. This estimate is based on applying "rate ratios" derived from an epidemiological study that compared risk factors among blacks and whites (Otten et al., 1990). The difference between the first and second rates represents the excess mortality of blacks that is related to lack of access to health care services.

Trends in the Data

The 1980 mortality rate from all causes for white males age 35 to 54 was 479.4 per 100,000 population; for same-age white females the rate was 250.3 per 100,000 (National Center for Health Statistics, 1980b). For black males between the ages of 35 and 54, death from all causes stood at 1,048 per 100,000 in 1980; for same-age black females the rate was 527.4 per 100,000. Based on these data, black men and women between the ages of 35 and 54 were 2.2 and 2.1 times more likely, respectively, than their white counterparts to have died in 1980.

By 1988 mortality rates for white males and females age 35 to 54 each had fallen 20 percent, to 381.6 per 100,000 for men and 200.7 per 100,000 for women. The corresponding death rate for black men was 948.4 per 100,000 (a 9.5 percent reduction compared with 1980); for black women the rate was 439.8 per 100,000 (a 16 percent reduction from the 1980 level).

Data on risk factors from the National Health and Nutrition Examination Survey I Epidemiologic Follow-up Study (NHEFS) have been used to calculate the mortality risk ratios of blacks and whites (Otten et al., 1990). The risk ratios were adjusted to remove the influence of six well-established risk factors: smoking, systolic blood pressure, cholesterol level, body-mass index, alcohol intake, and diabetes. In 1980, for men age 35 to 54, the adjusted black-white risk ratio was 1.6; for women of the same age the ratio was 2.3.

Performing the calculations outlined in the measurement section above yields a crude potentially access-related excess mortality rate for blacks (Figure 3-3). In 1980, for men age 35 to 54, the rate was 393 per 100,000. In other words, nearly 39 percent of all deaths among middle-aged black men that year may be attributable to problems in gaining access to the personal health care system. In 1980, for black women age 35 to 54, the access-related death rate was 298.1 per 100,000, accounting for 56 percent of all deaths in this group. These figures must be considered a crude rate at present. As suggested in the recommendations that follow, further research is needed to account for patient characteristics that are not measured by known risk factors.

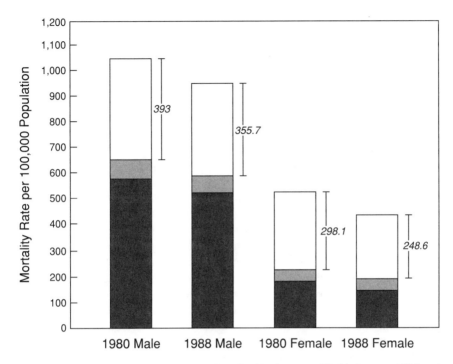

FIGURE 3-3 Estimated excess mortality for blacks, ages 35–54, by sex, 1980 and 1988. The areas indicated are the estimated mortality for blacks if age-specific mortality rates were equal to those of whites (■); the estimated excess black mortality due to differences in controllable risk factors (▨); and estimated excess black mortality due to differences in access to personal health care (☐). SOURCE: Calculated as described in the text above, under "Measuring the Indicator."

In 1988 it appears that the number of deaths among blacks attributable to access-related problems decreased for both men and women. For black men age 35 to 54, the rate was 355.7 per 100,000; for black women the rate was 248.6 per 100,000. These reductions reflect the overall decline in death rates for blacks and whites and are a continuation of the trend of previous decades. Although they have not been calculated, it is unlikely that the black-white risk ratios for 1988 differ substantially from those determined by Otten for the 1970s when the subjects were surveyed.

Because the calculation of relative risks relies on data from health examination surveys conducted in the 1970s, the drop in excess rates is due solely to changes in black mortality, not changes in risk factor adjustments. It would be desirable, therefore, to have more up-to-date data on risk factors.

Recommendations

Much of the interest in excess mortality has focused on clarifying the role of behavioral and environmental risk factors in producing it, with an eye to designing prevention strategies. More recently, researchers have begun to concentrate on what heretofore had been considered an unexplained residual statistic that now appears to be related to access to and quality of care. The committee believes that this residual deserves further investigation as a potential access measure that can be used in tandem with a better understanding of behavioral and physiological risk factors.

Determining access-related excess mortality raises a number of measurement issues that also deserve further investigation. As mentioned, the rate ratios that are used to adjust for the effect of a set of risk factors for the 1970s were used to calculate access-related excess mortality in 1988. Without new risk data, however, only part of the story can be revealed. Although they might be similar, the actual adjustment for 1988 would not be exactly the same as the adjustment for 1980. It is important to note that most of these risk factors are slow to change. Therefore, changes in risk factors probably have had only a modest effect on changes in death rates during this short period. Moreover, knowing about a change in one risk factor (lower smoking rates, for example) is not sufficient because it is the interaction of the six factors that drives the models.

The measurement of access-related excess mortality is also complicated by the fact that some of the risk factors used in the calculation can be thought of as early stages of disease. For instance, hypertension is an important risk factor for both heart disease and stroke, and it is a disease in itself. "Removing" its effect in an excess mortality calculation removes as well the possible impact that access to medical care earlier in life could have had in preventing hypertension.

Any approach such as this, in which the final result is based on a residual, assumes that appropriate statistical models and data exist to correctly and completely remove the effects of the non-access-related determinants of mortality. It further assumes that all variability in mortality rates that is not attributable to measurable, non-access-related factors is related to access—that is, that there is no "noise" in the data that is not related to risk factors or access. This conclusion cannot be drawn with any certainty.

The current approach does not specifically identify the impact of chronic disease on access-related excess mortality. A rough approximation of this impact, however, can be obtained by studying an age cohort in which the incidence of chronic disease is likely to be quite high (persons age 35 to 54). In addition, the approach does not distinguish those diseases for which access is an important predictor of death from those for which it is not. The impact of the use of health care services is likely to be much greater for diseases and conditions that are amenable to medical intervention than for those on which such services appear to have little influence (Poikolainen and Eskola, 1986).

The model used by the committee to adjust overall mortality rates to take into account risk factors for disease is an important first step in improving such calculations because it points to clear shortcomings in the available data. The committee believes that research on access-related excess mortality must begin to focus on specific diseases, particularly those amenable to access-related prevention services or amelioration. The present analysis would have been enhanced by the availability of data from a somewhat older age cohort in which chronic diseases were a higher fraction of all deaths. Even better would be data from patient cohorts with specific diseases. It would also be desirable to develop models that compare groups on the basis of factors other than race—for example, income and insurance status.

The National Mortality Followback Survey could be used to explore specific common causes of death related to problems of access. For example, a recent study used data from this survey to analyze differences in the age at death for uninsured and privately insured people between the ages of 25 and 64 who died of acute myocardial infarction (Hadley et al., 1992). This study found that the uninsured were about two years younger at the time of death and that they had significantly less access to care in the year before death (fewer physician visits, greater trouble securing a physician, fewer hospitalizations and hospital days). The investigators controlled for (i.e., "removed") the effects of differences in sex, race, marital status, income, and several risk factors associated with heart attacks. This research also revealed that for most causes of death there were too few cases under the age of 65 included in the followback survey to permit meaningful multivariate analysis. The value of the survey could be enhanced by limiting the number of causes of death surveyed and increasing the numbers of deaths sampled for each of those causes, or by increasing the size of the survey.

The CDC has experimented with a mortality followback pilot study in collaboration with six state diabetes control programs. Among other findings, the study revealed that high blood pressure was not being controlled in a substantial part of the population and that the rate of blood glucose monitoring was relatively low (Bild et al., 1988).

Whatever adjustment model is used, calculations of the risk ratios of blacks compared with whites and those of other ethnic groups (as well as income groups) must be conducted on a more timely basis. Unfortunately, the large-scale epidemiological studies needed to determine trends in excess mortality are too expensive and complex to be replicated every year. It may be possible to derive similar information using mortality rates and risk factor data available through the vital statistics system and regular surveys, such as the NHIS and the BRFSS. If reliable statistical risk models can be developed, using variables from these two sources but based on data sets like the NHEFS, current mortality rates and current risk factor data can be combined into annual estimates of excess mortality.

OBJECTIVE 5: REDUCING MORBIDITY AND PAIN THROUGH TIMELY AND APPROPRIATE TREATMENT

Utilization Indicator: Percentage of Healthy Individuals Who Do Not Contact a Physician During an Acute Episode of Illness

People who perceive themselves to be in good to excellent health occasionally have an acute illness or a flare-up of a chronic condition that causes them to temporarily limit their normal activities. This could mean staying home from work or school, being restricted to bed, or reducing one's normal activities for more than half a day. During these episodes, a person may believe that his or her symptoms warrant medical attention. Differences among subpopulations in the frequency with which they contact a physician during such episodes could reflect differences in access. Physician contacts refer to consultation either in person or by telephone with a physician or someone (e.g., nurse, physician's assistant) who is supervised by a physician. Data on physician contacts, perceived health status, and restricted activity days are available from the NHIS.

Roughly 800 million physician contacts are made each year by people believing themselves to be in good or excellent health. In addition to requiring treatment for acute care conditions and low-impact chronic conditions, many of these people have undetected chronic diseases that might be aided by prompt medical attention. For example, a 1987 NCHS study estimated that nearly 50 percent of diabetes cases in the United States from 1976 through 1980 went undiagnosed. This indicator contrasts with that for continuing care for chronic disease in that those individuals, perceiving themselves to be in poor health, are more likely to know that they require continuous medical monitoring and care.

Someone who feels ill enough to restrict his or her activities may not necessarily need to seek assistance from a health care provider. For example, many colds and cases of back pain are self-limiting, and the individual can resume normal activities after rest. Thus, choosing not to visit a physician for these conditions may be appropriate utilization. The point of the indicator, however, is that over a broad range of many people and providers, average utilization should not differ among groups by, for example, insurance status. Individual variation in under- and overutilization should be canceled out. In other words, differences among population groups can reflect the presence of access barriers or overuse by groups with high incomes or adequate insurance coverage. Because the measurement techniques for this indicator are not well developed, it is not possible to distinguish who may be overusing ambulatory care services. Nonetheless, it is important to monitor systematic differential rates of use by those potentially facing barriers to entering the personal health care system. The results of monitoring utilization must be interpreted in light of related outcome indicators (to follow) and investigated by research studies that explore the issues in greater depth.

Measuring the Indicator

The primary medical concern of the 90 percent of the population who see themselves as being in good health is whether they will be able to see a doctor when needed. This indicator attempts to measure this concern by singling out healthy people who suddenly become so sick that they must reduce their normal activities. The question is whether such characteristics as insurance status, income, and race have an effect on whether they obtain medical attention.

The committee used the NHIS to identify individuals who reported themselves to be in good to excellent health and who had had at least one day of restricted activity in the two weeks prior to being interviewed. Comparisons were then made among those who had potential access barriers.

Trends in the Data

Table 3-26 displays the proportion of healthy individuals who had *no* physician contacts during a period in which they reduced their activities because of health problems. The majority of people, regardless of whether they had insurance, did not contact a physician by phone or in person. However, people without insurance or Medicare recipients without supplementary policies were less likely than those with private insurance to seek medical care or advice. The differences range from 5 to 10 percentage points. The likelihood of contacting a physician decreases by about 5 percentage points at the lowest income levels both for the uninsured and privately insured, although the differences are not statistically significant. Future monitoring should be alert to signs of whether anticipated out-of-pocket costs are deterring some of the insured from obtaining services.

The committee's data analysis revealed only slight differences between blacks and whites on this indicator (Table 3-26). Uninsured blacks, for example, were about three percentage points more likely not to contact a physician than uninsured whites. The difference between Hispanics and non-Hispanics was also about three percentage points. A 1986 telephone survey documented similar small differences between whites and blacks in

TABLE 3-26 Percentage of Individuals in Good to Excellent Health Who Had No Physician Contact During Period of Restricted Activity

Insurance Status	Total	White	Black
Uninsured	66	65	68
Private health insurance	55	56	55
Medicaid only	54	53	59
Medicare only	60	57	*
Medicare and private health insurance	50	49	*

*Estimates for which the relative standard error exceeds 30 percent are not reported.

SOURCE: Unpublished data from the National Health Interview Survey, National Center for Health Statistics, 1989.

terms of their use of ambulatory care. A higher proportion of blacks (39.3 percent) than whites (33.4 percent) who rated themselves in good to excellent health had gone without an ambulatory care visit during the previous year. However, this survey illustrates the importance of probing further. Blacks' perceptions of the quality of ambulatory care differed significantly from those of whites. For example, 23.3 percent of blacks compared with 9 percent of whites, felt that their physician did not inquire sufficiently about pain; 44.2 percent of blacks, compared with 27.5 percent of whites, felt that their doctors did not adequately explain the seriousness of their illness or injury (Blendon et al., 1989).

Whether generally healthy people are able to see a physician during an acute episode of illness may be related to some extent to their relationship to the personal health care system for routine care. Analysis of the 1986 Robert Wood Johnson Foundation access survey revealed that not having a regular source of care was a risk factor for not receiving recommended medical care. This includes not only cancer screening (as noted in the discussion of a previous indicator) but also whether a person is likely to see a physician for serious medical symptoms such as chest pain during exercise, abnormal bleeding, or loss of consciousness. Survey items that investigate whether people have a "regular source of care" have been relied upon as a global indicator of "access to continuity of care"; however, methodological studies caution against overinterpreting these results because access barriers are only one reason why people may not have a regular source. For example, many people who have insurance and an adequate income nevertheless choose not to have a regular health care provider (Hayward et al., 1991b).

Data from the Hispanic Health and Nutrition Examination Survey (conducted from 1982 through 1984) on the use of health services among Hispanics shows that the frequency of physician visits differed markedly among the three major Hispanic groups living in the United States. Of those who were uninsured, Mexican Americans were three times more likely than Cuban Americans and nearly four times more likely than Puerto Ricans never to have had a routine physical examination (29.5 percent, 9.9 percent, and 7.7 percent, respectively). With the exception of those who had non-Medicare, non-Medicaid public insurance, Mexican Americans were also the least likely among all insured Hispanics to have ever had a physical examination (Trevino et al., 1991).

The 1988 NHIS Child Health Supplement found that a greater proportion of high-income children (92.4 percent for household incomes over $40,000) compared with low-income children (83.8 percent for incomes less than $10,000) had a source of routine medical care. This relationship was equally true when insurance status was taken into account. Insured children were much more likely than uninsured children to have a regular source of care (91.9 percent compared with 79 percent; Bloom, 1988).

Data from the 1982 preventive care supplement to the NHIS revealed a similar correlation among income, insurance status, and the use of routine health services by children age 5 through 16. Children in families with incomes below the poverty line were more likely than their wealthier counterparts to be either nonusers of routine physical, dental, and eye examinations or to be less frequent users of those services. Children with Medicaid were more likely than those without Medicaid or other third-party insurance to use one of the three services. This relationship was particularly strong for physical examinations: 82.7 percent of children with Medicaid, compared with 62.2 percent of those without it, had had such an exam (Newacheck and Halfon, 1988).

Recommendation

National Health Interview Survey Enhancements. In conjunction with efforts to improve monitoring of continuing care for chronic diseases, the NCHS should explore methods to better understand the timely and appropriate use of physician services during episodes of acute illness. Of particular interest are acute illnesses and early stages of chronic illness that have the potential for serious consequences if left untreated.

Utilization Indicator: Dental Services

Annual dental visits include all visits made to a dentist, or to a technician or hygienist under a dentist's supervision, for regular, specialized, or emergency dental care. Services such as mass screening at schools or other institutions are excluded.

People visit the dentist for many reasons: to have a regular oral examination and checkup, to receive preventive services (such as sealants and fluoride treatment), to obtain emergency treatment for pain, to receive fillings for decayed teeth, to have teeth extracted, or to receive fixed or removable appliances for missing teeth. Dental care can help resolve disease problems and improve functioning, such as the ability to eat and speak; it can also improve appearance. To the extent that dental care can prevent the loss of permanent teeth and help individuals maintain a healthy cosmetic dentition, it plays an important social role in communication and job performance.

There are other important reasons for tracking access to dental services. Since only about a third of Americans are covered by dental insurance, the use of dental services is quite sensitive to income. That is, those in higher-income brackets are more likely to visit a dentist than those less financially well off, regardless of broader health insurance coverage. This relationship has important implications for understanding access more broadly across the health care system.

Part of the committee's mandate was to consider access problems across a wide range of clinical areas. Dentistry constitutes a health service that nearly everyone needs but that is frequently overlooked as a segment of the personal health care system. In the future, in addition to dentistry, access monitoring activities should also focus on barriers to other types of health care, including that provided by nurses and allied health professionals.

Measuring the Indicator

Access to dental services is measured most commonly by the average number of dental visits per person per year. Data on dental visits come from supplements to the NHIS; the most recent NHIS data on dental services are from 1989. Yet the method falls short in two respects: it fails to distinguish differences in the content of visits, and it does not indicate the type, if any, of patient insurance. The poor and many of the uninsured often forgo routine preventive and restorative dental care. Thus, when dental problems become severe, they are more likely to require extractions instead of other more preferable, but expensive, procedures. A monitoring method must be able to disaggregate the content of dental visits to determine when the kind of dental care received is related to problems with access. To sort out the effects of financial barriers, it would be desirable to have more refined information about insurance coverage for dental services. Most surveys identify only those with private insurance, aggregating those with publicly funded insurance, such as Medicaid, and those with no insurance at all.

Trends in the Data

Table 3-27 displays the number of dental visits and percentage of the population that never visited a dentist according to selected patient characteristics. Between 1983 and 1989 the average number of dental visits per person in the United States increased 14 percent, from 1.8 to 2.1. During the same period, the proportion of those who had never visited a dentist fell

TABLE 3-27 Dental Visits, by Selected Patient Characteristics,[a] 1964, 1983, and 1989

Characteristics	Dental Visits			Never Visited Dentist		
	1964	1983	1989	1964	1983	1989
Total	1.6	1.8	2.1	15.5	7.7	6.4
Age (years)						
2–14	1.3	2.0	2.1	46.6	23.5	19.7
15–44	1.9	1.9	2.4	4.0	1.7	1.4
45–64	1.7	2.0	2.4	1.3	0.6	0.4
65 and over	0.8	1.5	2.0	1.5	0.9	0.5
Sex						
Male	1.4	1.7	2.0	16.1	7.9	6.7
Female	1.7	2.1	2.3	15.0	7.8	6.1
Race						
White	1.7	2.0	2.3	13.8	7.2	6.1
Black[b]	0.8	1.2	1.2	28.0	10.3	7.7
Family income[c]						
Less than $14,000	0.9	1.2	1.3	27.4	11.2	9.5
$14,000–$24,999	0.9	1.5	1.5	22.0	9.8	7.8
$25,000–$34,999	1.4	2.2	2.2	15.8	7.2	6.3
$35,000–$49,999	1.9	2.5	2.7	10.9	4.5	4.5
$50,000 or more	2.7	2.9	3.1	7.2	3.6	3.4
Location of residence						
Within MSA	1.8	2.1	2.2	14.4	7.2	6.2
Outside MSA	1.2	1.6	1.7	17.9	8.6	5.8

MSA, metropolitan statistical area.

[a]Gender, race, family income, and location of residence are age adjusted.

[b]Category of "black" in 1964 includes all nonwhite races.

[c]Family income categories are for 1989. Comparable income categories for 1964 are as follows: less than $2,000; $2,000–$3,999; $4,000–$8,999; and $10,000 or more. For 1983 the categories are less than $10,000; $10,000–$18,999; $19,000–$29,999; $30,000–$39,999; and $40,000 or more.

SOURCE: Unpublished data from the National Health Interview Surveys, National Center for Health Statistics, 1964, 1983, 1989.

from 7.7 percent to 6.4 percent. However, the black-white disparity in the use of dental services grew, as blacks remained at 1.2 visits per year and white usage increased to 2.3. Those over age 65 have markedly changed their use of dental services, increasing the average number of visits per year from 1.5 in 1983 to 2.0 in 1989. This continues a long-term trend that is related in part to greater numbers of the elderly retaining their teeth longer as they age.

Some indication of the benefit of increased dental visits and greater use of fluoride is apparent in the changing tooth decay experience of U.S. schoolchildren. Compared with the early 1970s, most children in the late 1980s experienced much less tooth decay and thus received fewer fillings and had fewer missing teeth. However, a significant minority of children still experience substantial tooth decay that will compromise their adult dentition if they do not gain access to primary dental care (Office of Technology Assessment, 1990).

Hispanic American adults seem to be at high risk for dental diseases. This group had twice the mean number of untreated decayed teeth of Hispanic children, indicating that lack of access to dental care extends into adult life. The result is that dentate Cuban American and Puerto Rican adults are missing about twice as many teeth as are white, non-Hispanic adults.

The prevalence of gingivitis is also higher among Hispanic Americans than among white non-Hispanics, as estimated during the 1985–1986 survey of employed American adults conducted by the National Institute of Dental Research. Hence, the higher incidence of dental diseases and the presence of high levels of untreated oral conditions suggest that Hispanic American adults experience problems in gaining access to dental care that can compromise the quality of their adult lives (Ismail and Szpunar, 1990).

Household income was directly related to the use of dental services (see Table 3-27). In 1989 people with incomes of more than $50,000 had an average of 3.1 dental visits per year, more than twice the average for those with incomes under $14,000. There was also a small but consistent difference in the number of annual visits made by those living in cities compared with those living outside a metropolitan area, suggesting that people in more rural communities may experience an access barrier.

Not having dental insurance appears to be an important access barrier to dental care. According to the 1986 NHIS, 37.8 percent of those interviewed had dental insurance. Whether one has dental coverage appears to depend on a number of sociodemographic characteristics, including age, race, income, education, and overall health status. For example, people age 25–54 were more likely than those older or younger to have coverage. Whites were more likely than blacks to have dental insurance (39.3 versus 28.4 percent, respectively), and men were slightly more likely than women to be insured (38.6 percent of men had coverage). Only 10 percent of those with incomes under $10,000 had dental insurance, compared with 56.6 percent of those with incomes above $35,000. People with more than a high school education were almost three times as likely as those with less than nine years of education to have dental insurance (44.6 versus 15.3 percent, respectively). Those in good to excellent health were nearly twice as likely as those in fair or poor health to have dental insurance (41.5 versus 23.4 percent, respectively).

In 1989 those with dental insurance made an average of about one more visit annually to the dentist than those without insurance (2.7 visits compared with 1.7 visits; Table 3-28). This same insurance-related differential was apparent for both blacks and whites. Regardless of insurance status, whites (2.8 visits by insured, 1.8 visits by uninsured) made more visits than blacks (1.7 visits by insured, 0.9 visits by uninsured). A factor of concern is that the use of dental services among blacks appeared to decline between 1986 and 1989. At each income level, those with insurance made more visits than those without insurance. It is not clear why those with insurance and incomes under $10,000 had such a high number of visits; it may relate to the fact that only a small percentage (10 percent) of this group has insurance.

The committee's analysis of hospital discharge data from 11 states revealed that residents in low-income zip codes are almost three times (2.86) as likely to be admitted to hospitals for dental conditions as those from high-income zip codes. Hospital admission for the specific set of ICD-9

TABLE 3-28 Annual Dental Visits, by Dental Insurance Status and Selected Characteristics, 1986 and 1989

Characteristic	Private Insurance		Uncovered	
	1986	1989	1986	1989
Total	2.6	2.7	1.7	1.7
Race				
Black	2.0	1.7	1.1	0.9
White	2.7	2.8	1.8	1.8
Family income				
Less than $10,000	2.9	2.1	1.2	1.2
$10,000–$19,999	1.9	2.1	1.5	1.3
$20,000–$34,999	2.6	2.3	2.1	1.8
$35,000 or more	2.9	3.1	2.4	2.5

SOURCE: Unpublished data from the National Health Interview Surveys, National Center for Health Statistics, 1986 and 1989.

codes selected by the committee is indicative of advanced dental disease that may be caused by lack of adequate ambulatory dental care. Because admission rates for dental problems are fairly low (less than 0.1 per 1,000 population for the 11 states studied), by itself the measure has limited utility as an outcome indicator.

Two recent studies have shown that Medicaid coverage of dental services appears to impose its own set of access problems on low-income patients. In a review of the Medicaid policies of seven states, the Office of Technology Assessment (1990) found significant differences in the dental services offered. To varying degrees, each state program failed to adequately cover a number of basic dental services. Several specific barriers to dental services were identified, including low Medicaid reimbursement rates, which resulted in inadequate treatment for patients or discouraged dentists from participating in the program; insufficient subsidization of patient transportation costs to the dentist's office; and Medicaid recipients' own lack of awareness of their dental benefits, failure to use their benefits even when aware of them, and negative perceptions about dentistry.

A study of California's Medi-Cal program (Damiano et al., 1990) found a similar set of problems. Medi-Cal reimbursement rates for dental services are significantly lower than the fees charged by private practitioners, which discourages many dentists from treating those covered by the program. Only about 15 percent of all general practice and pediatric dentists in the state accept new Medi-Cal patients; by geographic area, 28 of California's 58 counties had no dentists willing to accept Medi-Cal patients. Overall, the 1,800 dentists in Medi-Cal's dental referral program were responsible for meeting the needs of about 3 million eligible patients across the state.

Recommendations

NHIS Dental Supplements. Questions in future NHIS dental supplements should gather information not only about private insurance coverage but also about publicly funded coverage, such as that provided by Medicaid, Medicare (for oral surgery), the Department of Veterans Affairs, and the military (for dependents). The specific content of care received by patients, including preventive and routine checkups, restorative treatment, extractions, and full or partial dentures, should be captured by the survey. NHIS questions should also probe in greater detail the factors, including cost, that prevent patients from visiting the dentist.

Research Studies. The committee recommends that research be conducted to determine trends in the effect of private insurance on access to various types of dental services.

Outcome Indicator: Avoidable Hospitalization
for Acute Conditions

For the purposes of this indicator, hospitalizations are hospital admissions for conditions related to an acute episode of disease. Avoidable hospitalizations are those that probably would not have occurred had the patient received appropriate and timely outpatient (ambulatory) medical care.

People who are in good to excellent health—the population of interest in this objective—may seek medical attention for any number of reasons. (See the discussion for the indicator "Routine Physician Contacts" above.) The personal health care system in some cases provides only symptomatic relief to patients for conditions that would resolve independent of any medical intervention. In other situations, however, symptoms that are not addressed in a timely fashion can evolve into acute medical problems requiring hospitalization.

For example, a child with pain and fever may be treated by a parent with an over-the-counter cold medication. If the child is from a family with no regular source of medical care and if the symptoms become severe enough, a visit to the emergency room may become necessary. An emergency room physician, unaware that there has been a history of these infections, may release the child to his or her parents. At home the child may get progressively worse and eventually develop severe otitis media requiring hospitalization.

There are many other examples of potential problems faced by people without a regular source of medical care. Someone who experiences frequent urination, a burning sensation, or intermittent pain upon urination, indicating a relatively simple-to-treat urinary tract infection, may, if untreated, be at risk for developing a severe kidney infection. A persistent cough can signal any number of conditions, including tuberculosis or pneumonia. Untreated diarrhea can evolve into severe gastroenteritis.

For the significant segment of the population with no or inadequate health insurance, or who for other reasons have no regular source of medical care, hospital emergency rooms are increasingly being used as walk-in clinics for all manner of health complaints. Although few would maintain that the hospital emergency department is an optimum site for primary care, in the absence of a well-organized system of ambulatory care for those unable to afford private medical care, it is one of the only options. Unfortunately, especially in inner-city hospitals, inpatient bed space is limited. Many emergency rooms overflow not only with patients waiting to be seen by a doctor but also with patients who are already evaluated and are waiting to be assigned a hospital bed. Some evidence suggests that a significant proportion of emergency room patients with serious medical conditions leave the hospital without ever being seen. One of two recent studies found that

11 percent of such patients ended up being hospitalized within the next week (Baker et al., 1991). In the second study, only 4 percent ended up being hospitalized but 27 percent returned to an emergency room (Bindman et al., 1991).

Measuring the Indicator

The committee used the same approach to measure avoidable hospitalization for acute conditions that it used for chronic disease conditions (see Objective 3). The only difference is that a different set of ICD-9 diagnosis codes will be highlighted in the analysis.

The committee chose to examine acute-illness-related data for diagnoses that, with timely and effective outpatient care, normally would not result in a hospital admission. Mild cases of bacterial pneumonia, cellulitis, urinary tract infections, ENT (ear, nose, and throat) infections, and precursor infections leading to pelvic inflammatory disease can often be managed with antibiotics in outpatient settings, preventing the disease from becoming more severe. In selecting specific ICD-9 codes to represent ambulatory-care-sensitive conditions, an effort was made to screen out, where possible, those admissions that would cloud interpretation of the phenomenon of interest: timely and appropriate outpatient care. For example, cases of cellulitis in which a surgical procedure was performed are excluded, because they may be repeat hospitalizations for plastic surgery procedures or trauma cases. Admissions from nursing facilities were also excluded, since these cases have been under at least nominal medical care.

The committee recognizes that the causes behind many hospital admissions for acute conditions are more complex than a delayed outpatient visit. Higher rates of admissions from low-income neighborhoods may be due to lack of health knowledge, comorbidities, or differences in prevalence arising from environmental and social factors related to poverty—all of which can interact with financial barriers to delay care. However, differences in the prevalence of various diseases among the poor, while explaining some portion of admission rate differentials, do not obviate conclusions about the presence of access problems. To counterbalance social factors, equity of access to appropriate care may require more or different types of services for some populations. For instance, these services might include nutrition education for new mothers to lower rates of gastrointestinal diseases, screening young women for venereal disease to lower their rates of pelvic inflammatory disease, or addiction services for alcoholics who are at risk of various medical complications.

As in the previous indicators that use hospital discharge data, this indicator is measured by the ratio of hospital admissions from low-income zip codes to admissions from high-income zip codes. High-income areas are

TABLE 3-29 Ambulatory-Care-Sensitive Conditions: Acute Disease, 1988 Admission Rates by Zip Code Income Groupings, Nonelderly Population, 11 States

Condition	Low-Income Admissions/ 1,000 Population	High-Income Admissions/ 1,000 Population	Ratio, Low/ High Income
Bacterial pneumonia	4.39	0.81	5.42
Cellulitis	2.11	0.42	5.02
Dehydration as primary diagnosis	0.59	0.28	2.11
Gastroenteritis	1.30	0.68	1.91
Kidney/urinary infection	1.28	0.46	2.78
Severe ear, nose, and throat infections	0.82	0.24	3.42
Skin graft with cellulitis	0.46	0.08	5.75
Total	10.95	2.97	3.69

SOURCE: Joint data and analysis by the Codman Research Group, the Ambulatory Care Access Group (United Hospital Fund of New York), and the IOM Access Monitoring Committee.

those in which 10 percent or less of families have incomes below $15,000. In low-income areas, 60 percent or more of the families have incomes of $15,000 or less. Again, the focus is on those under 65 years of age.

Trends in the Data

Table 3-29 highlights a number of ambulatory-care-sensitive conditions relevant to the present discussion of hospitalization for acute disease that might have been avoided with timely and appropriate care. For most of the diagnoses in the table, the rates of hospital admissions from low-income zip codes were two to five times higher than rates from high-income zip codes. The overall average ratio was 3.69.

Recommendation

Many patients seen in a hospital emergency room may be unable or unwilling to do what is necessary to recuperate at home from a serious illness. In many cases, such patients have poor social support networks, may live in homes that are overcrowded or without heat, or may be unable to afford the necessities of life, such as food. Relatives of such a patient may have low-income jobs that make it difficult for them to stay home and provide needed care for the sick person or to pay for needed medications. For these and other reasons, physicians may be inclined to hospitalize low-income patients more frequently than high-income ones. Current data on hospitalization do not take into account the possibility that physicians may be using different standards to admit patients (Billings et al., 1991). However, Billings' analysis of New York City data did indicate that the severity of illness for patients from the poorest zip codes was equivalent to that of patients from the highest-income zip code.

As was true for chronic-disease-related conditions, the committee believes that more detailed studies of patients and of admitting physicians are needed. These studies should sort out the relative contributions of the various factors that lead to the hospitalization of people without a source of regular medical care. Use of hospital discharge data will be enhanced to the extent that specific diagnoses can be explored in greater depth to determine their utility as indicators of access problems.

REFERENCES

Alexander, G. R., Tompkins, M. E., Peterson, D. J., and Weiss, J. 1991. Source of bias in prenatal care utilization indices: Implications for evaluating the Medicaid expansion. *American Journal of Public Health* 81:1013-1016.

American Cancer Society. 1989. Cancer Statistics, 1989. *CA: A Cancer Journal for Clinicians* 39:3-20.

American College of Obstetricians and Gynecologists, Committee on Professional Standards. 1989. *Standards for Obstetric–Gynecological Services*, Seventh edition. Washington, D.C.: ACOG.

Baker, D. W., Stevens, C. D., and Brook, R. H. 1991. Patients who leave a public hospital emergency department without being seen by a physician. Causes and consequences. *Journal of the American Medical Association* 266:1085-1090.

Behrman, R. E. 1987. Premature births among back women. *New England Journal of Medicine* 317:763-765.

Bild, D., Geiss, L. S., Teutsch, S. M., et al. 1988. Sentinel health events surveillance in diabetes. *Journal of Clinical Epidemiology* 41:999-1006.

Billings, J., Zeitel, L., Lukomnik, J., et al. 1991. *Analysis of Variation in Hospital Admission Rates Associated with Area Income in New York City*. New York: Ambulatory Care Access Project/United Hospital Fund of New York.

Bindman, A. B., Grumbach, K., Keane, D., Rauch, L., and Luce, J. M. 1991. Consequences of queuing for care at a public hospital emergency department. *Journal of the American Medical Association* 266:1091-1096.

Blendon, R. J., Aiken, L. H., Freeman, H. E., and Corey, C. R. 1989. Access to medical care for black and white Americans. *Journal of the American Medical Association* 261:278-281.

Bloom, B. 1988. *Health Insurance and Medical Care: Health of our Nation's Children, United States*. Advance Data No. 188. Hyattsville, Md.: National Center for Health Statistics.

Boutwell, R. C., and Mitchell, J. B. 1991. Diffusion of new technologies in the Medicare population: Implications for patient access and program expenditures. Paper presented at a meeting of the Association for Health Services Research, San Diego, July 2.

Brook, R. H., and Lohr, K. N. 1986. Will we need to ration effective health care? *Issues in Science and Technology* 3(Fall):68-77.

Buehler, J. W., Stroup, D. F., Klaucke, D. N., and Berkelman, R. L. 1989. The reporting of race and ethnicity in the National Notifiable Diseases Surveillance System. *Public Health Reports* 104:457-465.

Caan, B., Horgen, D., Margen, S., King, J., and Jewell, N. 1987. Benefits associated with WIC supplemental feeding during the interpregnancy interval. *The American Journal of Clinical Nutrition* 45:29-41.

Centers for Disease Control. 1978. *CDC Analysis of Nutritional Indices for Selected WIC Participants.* Document No. FNS-176. Atlanta: Centers for Disease Control.

Centers for Disease Control. 1988. Progress in chronic disease prevention: Screening for cervical and breast cancer—Southeastern Kentucky. *Morbidity and Mortality Weekly Report* 36:845-849.

Centers for Disease Control. 1989a. Behavioral risk factor surveillance—Selected states, 1987. *Morbidity and Mortality Weekly Report* 38:469-473.

Centers for Disease Control. 1989b. National Infant Mortality Surveillance (NIMS), 1980. *Morbidity and Mortality Weekly Report*—CDC Surveillance Summaries, Vol. 38, No. SS-3. Atlanta: Centers for Disease Control.

Centers for Disease Control. 1989c. Summaries of notifiable diseases in the United States, 1989. *Morbidity and Mortality Weekly Report* 38:1-49.

Centers for Disease Control. 1990. Use of mammography—United States, 1990. *Morbidity and Mortality Weekly Report* 39:621-629.

Chorba, T. L., Berkelman, R. L., Safford, S. K., Gibbs, N. P., and Hull, H. F. 1990. Mandatory reporting of infectious diseases by clinicians. *Morbidity and Mortality Weekly Report* 39:1-17.

Cohen, D. A. 1991. Congenital syphilis. *New England Journal of Medicine* 324:1063-1064.

Cohen, D. A., Boyd, D., Prabhudas, I., and Mascola, L. 1990. The effects of case definition in maternal screening and reporting criteria on rates of congenital syphilis. *American Journal of Public Health* 80:316-317.

Coit, D. 1977. *WIC Program Prenatal Data Report.* Sacramento: California Department of Health Services.

Collins, T. R., DeMellier, S. T., Leeper, J. D., and Milo, T. 1985. Supplemental Food Program: Effects on health and pregnancy outcome. *Southern Medical Journal* 78:551-555.

Culpepper, L. 1991. *Reducing Infant Mortality: The Research Gaps.* Washington, D.C.: Health Resources and Services Administration.

Damiano, C., Brown, R., Johnson, J. D., and Scheetz, J. P. 1990. Access to dental care for Medi-Cal recipients. *California Policy Seminar Brief* 2(8) June.

Dorfman, D., and Glaser, J. H. 1990. Congenital syphilis present in infants after the newborn period. *New England Journal of Medicine* 323:1299-1301.

Drury, T. F., Harris, M., and Lipsett, L. F. 1981. Prevalence and management of diabetes. *Health, United States, 1981.* Washington, D.C.: U.S. Government Printing Office.

Food Research Action Center. 1991. *WIC: A Success Story* 3rd ed. Washington, D.C.: FRAC.

Fullilove, R. E., Thompson, M. T., Bowser, B. P., and Gross, S. A. 1990. Risk of sexually transmitted disease among black adolescent crack users in Oakland and San Francisco, Calif. *Journal of the American Medical Association* 263:851-855.

Gittelsohn, A. M., Halpern, J., and Sanchez, R. L. 1991. Income, race, and surgery in Maryland. *American Journal of Public Health* 81:1435-1441.

Greenberg, E. R., Chute, C. G., Stukel, T., et al. 1988. Special article: Social and economic factors in the choice of lung cancer treatment—A population-based study in two rural states. *New England Journal of Medicine* 318:612-617.

Hadley, J., Steinberg, E. P., and Feder, J. 1991. Comparison of uninsured and privately insured hospital patients. *Journal of the American Medical Association* 265:374-379.

Hadley, J., Steinberg, E., and Klag, M. 1992. *A Comparison of Insured Versus Uninsured Individuals Who Died from Acute Myocardial Infarction.* Washington, D.C.: Georgetown University Center for Health Policy.

Harlan, L. C., Bernstein, A. B., and Kessler, L. G. 1991. Cervical cancer screening: Who is not screened and why? *American Journal of Public Health* 81:885-890.

Hayward, R. S., Steinberg, E. P., Ford, D. E., Roizen, M. F., and Roach, K. W. 1991a. Preventive care guidelines: 1991a. *Annals of Internal Medicine* 114:758-783.

Hayward, R. A., Bernard, A. M., Freeman, H. E., and Corey, C. R. 1991b. Regular source of ambulatory care and access to health services. *American Journal of Public Health* 81:434-438.

Hinman, A. R. 1990. Immunizations in the U.S. *Pediatrics* 86(6, pt. 2, Suppl.):1064-1066.

Hinman, A. R. 1991. What will it take to fully protect all American children with vaccines? *American Journal of Diseases of Children* 145:559-562.

Institute of Medicine. 1985. *Preventing Low Birthweight.* Washington, D.C.: National Academy Press.

Institute of Medicine. 1988. *Prenatal Care—Reaching Mothers, Reaching Infants.* Washington, D.C.: National Academy Press.

Institute of Medicine. 1991. *Kidney Failure and the Federal Government.* R. A. Rettig and N. G. Levinsky, eds. Washington, D.C.: National Academy Press.

International Agency for Research on Cancer, Working Group on Evaluation of Cervical Cancer Screening Programmes. 1986. Screening for squamous cervical cancer: Duration of low risk after negative results of cervical cytology and its implication for screening policies. *British Medical Journal* 293:659-664.

Ismail, A. I., and Szpunar, S. M. 1990. The prevalence of total tooth loss, dental caries, and periodontal disease among Mexican Americans, Cuban Americans, and Puerto Ricans: Findings from HANES 1983-84. *American Journal of Public Health* 80(Suppl.):66-70.

Kennedy, E. T., and Kotelchuck, M. 1984. The effect of WIC supplemental feeding on birth weight: A case-control analysis. *The American Journal of Clinical Nutrition* 40:579-585.

Koss, L. G. 1989. The Papanicolaou test for cervical cancer detection. *Journal of the American Medical Association* 261:737-743.

Kotelchuck, M., Schwartz, J., Anderka, M., and Finison, K. 1984. Massachusetts Department of Public Health, Division of Family Services. WIC participation and pregnancy outcomes: Massachusetts statewide evaluation project. *American Journal of Public Health* 74:1086-1092.

Li, D-K., Ni, H., Schwartz, S. M., and Daling, J. R. 1990. Secular change in birthweight among Southeast Asian immigrants to the United States. *American Journal of Public Health* 80:685-688.

Lieberman, E., Ryan, K. J., Monson, R. R., and Schoenbaum, S. 1987. Risk factors accounting for racial differences in the rate of premature birth. *New England Journal of Medicine* 317:743-748.

Makuc, D. M., Freid, V. M., and Kleinman, J. C. 1989. National trends in the use of preventive health care by women. *American Journal of Public Health* 79:21-26.

McLaughlin, M., Wilkes, M., Blum, S., Hermoso, A., Schmid, G. 1989. Risks associated with acquiring chancroid genital ulcerative disease and HIV infection: A case control study. Paper presented at the Fifth International Conference on AIDS in Montreal, Canada, June 4–9.

Miller, C. A., Fine, A., and Adams-Taylor, S. 1989. *Monitoring Children's Health: Key indicators*, 2nd ed. Washington, D.C.: American Public Health Association.

Nanda, D., Feldman, J., Delke, I., Chintalapally, S., and Minkoff, H. 1990. Syphilis among parturients at an inner city hospital: Association with cocaine use and implications for congenital syphilis rates. *N.Y. State Journal of Medicine* 90:488-490.

National Cancer Institute. 1990a. *Cancer Statistics Review, 1973-1987*. L. A. G. Ries, B. F. Hankey, and B. K. Edwards, eds. NIH Pub. No. 90-2789. Bethesda, Md.: NCI.

National Cancer Institute, Breast Cancer Screening Consortium. 1990b. Screening mammography: A missed opportunity? Results of the NCI Breast Cancer Screening Consortium and National Health Interview Survey studies. *Journal of the American Medical Association* 264:54-58.

National Center for Health Statistics. 1980a. Comparability of reporting between the birth certificate and the National Natality Survey. Prepared by L. J. Querec. *Vital and Health Statistics*, Series 2, No. 83/G. DHEW Pub. No. (PHS) 80-1357. Washington, D.C.: U.S. Government Printing Office.

National Center for Health Statistics. 1980b. *Health, United States, 1980*. Washington, D.C.: U.S. Government Printing Office.

National Center for Health Statistics. 1983. Birth certificate completion procedures and the accuracy of Missouri birth certificate data. Prepared by G. Land and B. Vaughan. In: *Priorities in Health Statistics: Proceedings of the 19th National Meeting of the Public Health Conference on Records and Statistics*. Hyattsville, Md.: U.S. Department of Health and Human Services.

National Center for Health Statistics. 1987. Prevalence of Diagnosed Diabetes, Undiagnosed Diabetes, and Impaired Glucose Tolerance in Adults 20-74 Years of Age, United States, 1976-80. W. C. Hadden and M. I. Harris. *Vital and Health Statistics*. Series 11, No. 237. DHHS Pub. No. (PHS) 87-1687. Washington, D.C.: U.S. Government Printing Office.

National Center for Health Statistics. 1988. *Health Aspects of Pregnancy and Childbirth, United States, 1982—Data from the National Survey of Family Growth*. Series 23, No. 16. Hyattsville, Md.: U.S. Department of Health and Human Services.

National Center for Health Statistics. 1990a. Advanced Report of Final Natality Statistics, 1988. *Monthly Vital Statistics Report*, Vol. 39, No. 7(Suppl.). Hyattsville, Md.: U.S. Department of Health and Human Services.

National Center for Health Statistics. 1990b. Annual Summary of Births, Marriages, Divorces, and Deaths. *Monthly Vital Statistics Report*, Vol. 39, No. 13. Hyattsville, Md.: U.S. Department of Health and Human Services.

National Center for Health Statistics. 1990c. *Health, United States, 1990*. Washington, D.C.: U.S. Government Printing Office.

National Center for Health Statistics. 1991. The 1988 National Maternal and Infant Health Survey: Design, content, and data availability. M. Sanderson, P. J. Placek, and K. G. Keppel. *Birth* 18:26-32.

National Vaccine Advisory Committee. 1991. The measles epidemic: The problems, barriers, and recommendations. *Journal of the American Medical Association* 266:1547-1552.

Newacheck, P. W., and Halfon, N. 1988. Preventive care used by school-aged children: Differences by socioeconomic status. *Pediatrics* 82:462-468.

Office of Technology Assessment. 1988. *Healthy Children: Investing in the Future*. Washington, D.C.: U.S. Government Printing Office.

Office of Technology Assessment. 1990. *Children's Dental Services Under the Medicaid Program—Background Paper*. Washington, D.C.: U.S. Government Printing Office.

Otten, M. W., Teutsch, S. M., Williamson, D. F., and Marks, J. S. 1990. The effect of known risk factors on the excess mortality of black adults in the United States. *Journal of the American Medical Association* 263:845-850.

Poikolainen, K., and Eskola, J. 1986. The effect of health services on mortality: Decline in death rates from amenable and non-amenable causes in Finland, 1969-81. *Lancet* 1(8474): 199-202.

Pope, G. C. 1988. Medical conditions, health status, and health services utilization. *Health Services Research* 22:857-876.

Public Health Service Expert Panel on the Content of Prenatal Care. 1989. *Caring for our future: The Content of Prenatal Care.* Washington, D.C.: U.S. Public Health Service.

Rolfs, R. T., and Nakashima, A. K. 1990. Epidemiology of primary and secondary syphilis in the United States, 1981 through 1989. *Journal of the American Medical Association* 264:1432-1437.

Rosenbaum, S., Layton, C., and Liu, J. 1991. *The Health of American Children.* Washington, D.C.: Children's Defense Fund.

Rush, D., Alvir, J. M., Kenny, D. A., Johnson, S. S., and Horvitz, D. G. 1988a. Historical study of pregnancy outcomes. *The American Journal of Clinical Nutrition* 48:412-428.

Rush, D., Sloan, N. L., Leighton, J., Alvir, J. M., Horvitz, D. G., Seaver, W. B., et al. 1988b. Longitudinal study of women. *The American Journal of Clinical Nutrition* 48:439-483.

Schramm, W. 1986. Prenatal participation in WIC related to Medicaid costs for Missouri newborns: 1982 update. *Public Health Reports* 101:607-615.

Schulte, J. M., Bown, G. R., Zetzman, M. R., Schwartz, B., Green, H. G., Haley, C. E., et al. 1991. Changing immunization referral patterns among pediatricians and family practice physicians, Dallas County, Texas, 1988. *Pediatrics* 87:204-207.

Schwarcz, S. K., Bolan, G. A., Fullilove, M., McCright, J., and Kohn, R. 1989. Crack cocaine as a risk factor for gonorrhea among black teenagers. Paper presented at the 117th Annual Meeting of the American Public Health Association, Chicago, October 2–26.

Scribner, R., and Dwyer, J. H. 1989. Acculturation and low birthweight among Latinos in the Hispanic HANES. *American Journal of Public Health* 79:1263-1267.

Stoto, M. 1992. Premature Adult Mortality in Developed Countries: From Description to Explanation. Paper presented at a meeting of the International Union for the Scientific Study of Population, Taormina, Italy, June 1992. London: Oxford University Press.

Trevino, F. M., Moyer, M. E., Valdez, R. B., and Stroup-Benham, C. A. 1991. Health insurance coverage and utilization of health services by Mexican Americans, mainland Puerto Ricans, and Cuban Americans. *Journal of the American Medical Association* 265:233-237.

U.S. Department of Agriculture. 1987. *Estimation of Eligibility for the WIC Program.* Washington, D.C.

U.S. Department of Agriculture, Food and Nutrition Service. 1990. *The Savings in Medicaid Costs for Newborns and Their Mothers from Prenatal Participation in the WIC Program.* Princeton, N.J.: Mathematica Policy Research.

U.S. Department of Health and Human Services. 1986. *Report of the Secretary's Task Force on Black and Minority Health,* Vol. 7, Chemical Dependency and Diabetes. Washington, D.C.: U.S. Government Printing Office.

U.S. Department of Health and Human Services. 1991. *International Classification of Diseases, 9th revision, Clinical Modification,* 4th ed. DHHS Pub. No. PHS 91-1260. Washington, D.C.: U.S. Government Printing Office.

U.S. Preventive Services Task Force. 1989. *Guide to Clinical Preventive Services.* Baltimore: Williams & Wilkins.

U.S. Public Health Service. 1991. *Healthy People: National Health Promotion and Disease Prevention Objectives.* DHHS Pub. No. (PHS) 91-50212. Washington, D.C.: U.S. Government Printing Office.

Wenneker, M. B., and Epstein, A. M. 1989. Racial inequalities in the use of procedures for patients with ischemic heart disease in Massachusetts. *Journal of the American Medical Association* 261:253-257.

Wenneker, M. B., Weissman, J. S., and Epstein, A. M. 1990. The association of payer with utilization of cardiac procedures in Massachusetts. *Journal of the American Medical Association* 264:1255-1260.

Williams, B. C. 1990. Immunization coverage among preschool children: The United States and selected European countries. Child health in 1990: The United States compared to Canada, England and Wales, France, the Netherlands, and Norway. *Pediatrics* 86(Suppl.):1052-1056.

Wood, D. L., Hayward, R. A., Corey, C. R., Freeman, H. E., Shapiro, M. F. 1990. Access to medical care for children and adolescents in the United States. *Pediatrics* 86:666-673.

Zeitel, L., Bauer, T. A., and Brooks, P. 1991. *Infants at Risk: Solutions Within Our Reach.* New York: United Hospital Fund of New York/Greater New York Chapter of the March of Dimes.

4

Future Indicators

Given its limited time and resources, the IOM committee could not address all of the access problems that it would have liked to include in its report. The indicators described in the previous chapter constitute a first effort at balancing the constraints of offering a manageable set of social indicators on the one hand with the desire to represent a broad range of personal health services across the age continuum on the other. Because this baseline report merely sets the stage for continued monitoring, it is anticipated that future adjustments will be made in this basic set by expanding its breadth—not only through refinements in the ways that indicators are measured.

The purpose of this chapter is to present the committee's thinking about important directions for possible additions to the existing set of indicators. Individually, the topics represent access problems that are no less important a priority than those chosen for discussion in Chapter 3. These topics require further exploration because, to a greater or lesser degree, the state of the art of measuring them as an access problem is underdeveloped or because it is unclear whether routine data related to them will be available to track utilization or outcomes.

Box 4-1 lists the indicator topics that the committee has identified for future development. The topics were raised in the context of committee discussion either as concerns about access to a particular type of personal health service that had been omitted from the basic list or as concerns about a potentially vulnerable population group or a disease category. It is clear, however, that almost any access problem can be characterized on all three of these dimensions. (For example, there are substance abusers who require drug treatment services for their addictive disorders.) Moreover, as Aday (in press) has pointed out, many of the vulnerable populations whose access concerns us as a society have crosscutting needs. For instance, the broad group of alcohol and substance abusers can include high-risk mothers with fetal alcohol syndrome, intravenous drug users with AIDS, mentally ill substance abusers, drug users who attempt suicide, addictive families suffering domestic abuse, homeless people with substance abuse problems, and substance-abusing refugees.

Once a topic has been selected, the major challenge is to conceptualize an identifiable personal health service to serve as a utilization indicator and as an outcome measure that can be related to use or lack of use. The best utilization indicators are those for which there is a fairly well-recognized service intervention with clear guidelines regarding who should receive the service. Good outcome measures must be more than prevalence or incidence rates; they must reveal something about access. The best example is the incidence of a vaccine-preventable disease such as measles. In contrast, the incidence of colds would be difficult to relate to problems in access.

Once past the conceptual stage, it is necessary to identify a source of routine data. Potential data bases must be explored and the quality of the information assessed. As with the indicators in the initial monitoring set, a variety of problems involving data collection frequency, availability, and disaggregation must be confronted.

To illustrate the kind of analysis required, the committee commissioned papers on four of the topics: AIDS, substance abuse, and migrants and the homeless (Appendixes A–C). In fact, these papers go beyond illustration to provide the first strategic steps toward developing access monitoring indicators in these areas of interest.

BOX 4-1 Future Indicator Topics

HIV/AIDS*	People with disabilities
Substance abuse*	Family violence
Migrants*	Emergency services
Homeless people*	Post-acute-care services for the elderly
	Prescription drugs

*See Appendixes A, B, and C.

ACCESS TO HEALTH CARE
FOR PEOPLE WITH DISABILITIES

Disabilities as an issue affect every community, neighborhood, and family. Estimates of prevalence vary according to one's definition. A recent IOM report (1991), *Disability in America*, wrestled with the definitions and concepts surrounding systematic inquiry in this area. As an indication of general orders of magnitude, about 35 million Americans—one person in seven—have physical or mental impairments that interfere with their daily activities. More than 9 million disabled persons have functional limitations so severe that they cannot work, attend school, or maintain a household.

Disabled persons have become a focus of concern with regard to equity of access because of growing understanding about how insurance and other financial barriers are affecting them. Exclusion waivers for those with preexisting health conditions, higher premiums, and denials are ever-present phenomena of the health insurance industry—factors that hit those with disabilities particularly hard. An analysis of the 1984 National Health Interview Survey (NHIS) estimated that 11 percent of the 22.2 million people who are limited in their performance of major activities do not have insurance. The proportion of people with disabilities who rely on public programs is larger than that of the general population. Although the problem of denial of coverage as a consequence of being termed "medically uninsurable" is not well documented quantitatively, it is clear that employment does not guarantee health insurance coverage. Moreover, health insurance often does not cover the types of services that prevent disabling conditions from worsening or that improve functional ability. The lack of access to services that promote community care may foster greater use of institutionalization than is necessary. Because of the inadequacies of private health insurance, it is believed that a substantial number of disabled persons are forced to obtain supplemental security income or social security disability insurance in order to have health insurance coverage.

The current set of indicators captures one dimension of disability in its measurement of the use of physician services by those in poor to fair health. However, many other disabled individuals are in good to excellent health despite their limitations. Although these individuals can be identified by the NHIS, the utilization issue of particular relevance to future access monitoring involves those services related to the fact of being disabled. A variety of policy-relevant research questions have been asked in this vein—for example, to what services should persons with disability have access? The answer depends at least partly on the costs of such services relative to their benefits and the quality issue of how outcomes should be measured.

These factors cannot be readily translated into indicators. For one thing, caring for persons with disabilities involves more than personal health care services, with the lines between social and health services often be-coming blurred. It is generally believed that the character of these services and how they are organized make a difference for outcome; specifically, they need to be comprehensive, coordinated, and family centered. Those outcomes will most likely be measured in terms of quality of life and the prevention of secondary disabling disease conditions.

Enactment of the Americans with Disabilities Act further inspired the growing desire by policymakers and researchers to have better and more objective data on disabilities. During the course of the IOM Access Moni-toring Project, the National Center for Health Statistics was formulating plans to conduct a 1993–1994 supplement to the NHIS that focused on the noninstitutionalized disabled population. This survey should provide an opportunity to clarify definitions and measurement tools that would be in-strumental in developing a practical access indicator for disability.

FAMILY VIOLENCE

The inclusion of a separate chapter on violent and abusive behavior in the publication *Healthy People 2000* (U.S. Public Health Service, 1991) reflects a growing recognition of the problem as one that must be addressed not only by the legal, educational, and social welfare systems but by the health care system as well. The rubric of violent and abusive behavior can include the term "family violence," referring to child abuse, spousal abuse (especially battered women), and elder abuse.

Progress in developing an access indicator for this problem depends on identifying a generally agreed-upon personal health service that should be available to all who are at risk. For example, one of the *Healthy People 2000* objectives calls for the nation to "increase to at least 30 the number of states in which at least 50 percent of the children identified as neglected or physically or sexually abused receive physical and mental evaluation with appropriate followup as a means of breaking the intergenerational cycle of abuse." There are few patient outcome studies on the impact of medical interventions for battered women, but it seems clear that, at a minimum, referral to supportive services outside the personal health care system ought to be part of a standard of care.

Another facet of developing an indicator must be consideration of the potential barriers to access to services and how they might be measured. For example, battering is a major factor in illness and injury among women, but it is often overlooked by medical professionals. Some studies have shown that between 17 and 25 percent of all emergency department visits involve battered women, but emergency care providers typically identify less than 5 percent of the women with injuries or illnesses suggestive of abuse (McLeer and Anwar, 1989). In fact, the majority of battering-related illnesses and injuries are nontraumatic and are likely to be seen in primary care settings (Stark, 1981). The Lack of provider education and the absence of institutional protocols in delivery sites such as emergency rooms interfere with recognition of domestic violence as a medical problem and consequently preclude access to needed services. Moreover, access to health care for battered women is often controlled by their abusers; this is a structural barrier that prevents access to needed services. Financial and personal or cultural barriers to obtaining services also must be explored to determine whether they create inequities among subgroups in the population.

EMERGENCY SERVICES

Emergency services are a vital aspect of access. All groups, middle class as well as indigent, want to know that such services are available if needed and that they will function quickly and effectively. A report on access should tell citizens how well those who experience trauma and medical emergencies are likely to be served.

The minimum elements of an emergency medical system include the prehospital phase (e.g., a communications system, ambulances, helicopters, emergency medical personnel trained at various levels) and different categories of emergency departments, from hospitals that can stabilize and transfer patients to those that provide definitive care. A study by West et al. (1988) revealed that only two states had all components and statewide coverage of the eight essential components of a regional trauma system based on criteria set forth by the American College of Surgeons.

Any effort to develop an indicator of access to emergency care must begin by specifying performance measures that could indicate timeliness (e.g., response times) and effectiveness (e.g., mortality). Consideration must also be given to whether data bases exist to apply performance measures in reliable and valid ways. Because emergency systems are organized either locally or on a statewide basis, geographic comparisons would be required. It is possible that response times in poor neighborhoods may not be as fast as those in higher-income areas, creating an equity problem that should be measured at the individual or zip code level. Differing patterns of emergency department use by income and issues of inappropriate transfer among hospitals also raise questions about equity that might be monitored.

POST-ACUTE-CARE SERVICES FOR THE ELDERLY

Systemwide utilization data to track the elderly through parts of the health care system are not readily available (Densen, 1987). Questions that have been raised include the following: Under what conditions does a person receive a range of home health services versus being admitted to a nursing home? How can one conceptualize and measure the effect of access barriers on who receives what types of postacute services?

The National Medical Care Expenditure Survey confirmed what other surveys of the impaired elderly have found: in general, there are low levels of use of formal home and community services (Short and Leon, 1990). Home care, the most commonly used service, was used regularly by only 19.7 percent of those over 65 with functional difficulties. Whether low levels of use reflect the need for services, or financial barriers, or a lack of local resources is open to further research, according to the authors. Among those who use these services, however, having private insurance coverage in addition to Medicare did not make a difference in use. In addition, although differences were apparent in levels of use by region of the country, residence in a densely populated area did not affect the use of home care.

Developing an access indicator for home care and other types of long-term care will require better understanding of the characteristics that define a need for these services. To detect equity problems, it will be necessary first to classify people at risk according to their functional status, resource availability, and living arrangements so that the effects of financial and other access barriers can be measured. To date, most data on the use of these services have been available only through special surveys. A mechanism for regular reporting would be required to track access over time.

PRESCRIPTION DRUGS

From 1982 to 1988 prescription drug prices were the highest-inflated component of the health care sector. Today, in comparison, their share of the rapidly growing burden of health care expenditures has begun to shrink, although it is still sizable. On the one hand, third-party payment has grown to surpass out-of-pocket payment as the major revenue source for prescriptions (Schondelmeyer and Thomas, 1990). On the other hand, those who are uninsured or underinsured are likely to have an increasingly difficult time meeting these costs. This problem was a major motivation behind passage of a drug benefit in the Medicare Catastrophic Coverage Act of 1988 (P.L. 100-360). Analysis of data from the National Medical Care Expenditure Survey shows that Medicare beneficiaries without supplemental private insurance are about 10 percent more likely not to have had a drug prescribed than those with insurance (Moeller and Mathiowetz, 1989).

Conceptually, the major rationale for developing an indicator for access to prescription drugs would be to gain greater insight into the problems of those who may be able to see a physician but who do not follow the prescribed course of drug therapy. The hypothesis would be that lack of insurance, income, or both prevents the patient from purchasing prescribed medications. The inability to maintain a drug regimen could be the intervening mechanism that explains why some patients with chronic disease contribute to high rates of hospital admission for the ambulatory-care-sensitive conditions in the committee's primary list of indicators (Moeller and Mathiowetz, 1989).

REFERENCES

Aday, L. A. In press. *Health and Health Care of Vulnerable Populations.* San Francisco: Jossey-Bass.

Densen, P. 1987. The elderly and the health care system: Another perspective. *Milbank Quarterly* 65:614-638.

Institute of Medicine. 1991. *Disability in America: Toward a National Agenda for Prevention.* A. H. Pope and A. R. Tarlov, eds. Washington, D.C.: National Academy Press.

McLeer, S. V., and Anwar, R. 1989. A study of battered women in an emergency department. *American Journal of Public Health* 79:65-66.

Moeller, J. F., and Mathiowetz, N. 1989. Prescribed Medicines: A Summary of Use and Expenditures by Medicare Beneficiaries. National Medical Expenditure Survey, Research Findings No. 3. Washington, D.C.: Agency for Health Care Policy and Research.

Schondelmeyer, S., and Thomas, J. 1990. Trends in retail prescription expenditures. *Health Affairs* 9:131-145.

Short, P. F., and Leon, J. 1990. Use of Home and Community Services by Persons Ages 65 and Older with Functional Difficulties. National Medical Expenditure Survey, Research Findings No. 5. Washington, D.C.: Agency for Health Care Policy and Research.

Stark, E. 1981. Wife abuse in the medical setting: An introduction for health personnel. Monograph No. 7. Washington, D.C.: U.S. Department of Health and Human Services.

U.S. Public Health Service. 1991. *Healthy People: National Health Promotion and Disease Prevention Objectives.* DHHS Pub. No. (PHS) 91-50212. Washington, D.C.: U.S. Government Printing Office.

West, J. G., Williams, M. J., Trunkey, D. D., and Wolferth, C. C., Jr. 1988. Trauma systems, current status—Future challenges. *Journal of the American Medical Association* 259:3597-3600.

5

Recommendations

The purpose of this report is to lay a foundation for monitoring access to personal health care services. This effort, which by design has been limited in its focus, should be viewed as a first step toward developing a comprehensive set of national access indicators. Before presenting a compilation of the recommendations dispersed throughout the text, a set of crosscutting recommendations is offered to place the detailed recommendations in context.

RECOMMENDATIONS

Crosscutting Recommendations

The recommendations that follow are intended to improve the state of the art of monitoring, rather than provide explicit guidance on policies for financing medical care or delivering medical services. They arise out of the committee's general review of the indicators, trends in the data, measurement issues, and methodological problems involved in developing an access monitoring system.

State and Local Monitoring

States and local communities would benefit from a national access monitoring process. At the national level, the utilization and outcome indicators selected for this report are intended to be sensitive to the direction and extent of change in structural, financial, and personal barriers. At the state and local levels, these barriers are increasingly more definable in terms of a specific set of Medicaid benefits, institutional providers, population demographics, and physical features of the environment. (The advantage of proximity is being able to relate changes to more concrete circumstances.) However, local data are often incomplete, and resources may be insufficient to analyze the local data that do exist. The first step in addressing this problem is to identify clearly what data are needed (i.e., develop a monitoring framework) and how the data might be interpreted and then implement a cost-effective strategy for obtaining missing data.

The committee has proposed a framework for monitoring access and has analyzed specific indicators, demonstrating how they might be related to barriers. As a first step, in instances in which local data exist, states and localities can compare themselves with the national averages. They can also use additional data (such as those in surveys intended to determine which physicians accept Medicaid) and their general familiarity with the contours of the local health care system to draw conclusions about access problems faced by their vulnerable populations. In addition, an understanding of what can be done with the data will contribute to decisions about whether to invest in new data collection. Understanding the potential payoffs and the extent to which emerging national trends apply to local circumstances will allow communities to determine their needs for data collection.

The committee recognizes that constrained state and local public health budgets are likely to limit investment in major new surveys, hospital discharge systems, and cancer registries. To the extent that research and development costs can be borne by the federal government or by private foundations, the cost of implementing enhanced data systems could be reduced for local jurisdictions.

The Federal Role

Recommendation. The committee recommends that there be a federal organization responsible for monitoring access to personal health care services. This ongoing function should include the central collection, analysis, improvement, and dissemination of information on changes in access. The same organization should be responsible for providing technical assistance and consultation to local organizations that wish to conduct their own analyses of access indicators. This assistance will include activities to encourage improved technical capacity and, where appropriate, to promote consistent definitions and analytic approaches.

It was beyond the scope of the IOM committee's charge to identify precisely what entity in the government or private sector should have continuing responsibility for both monitoring access to health care and improv-

ing the state of the art. However, the committee agreed that overall responsibility should be assigned to the U.S. Department of Health and Human
Services. The challenge for the Secretary of Health and Human Services
will be to delegate authority to the appropriate agency within the department to ensure an institutionalization of the monitoring function.

In the past, the following criteria (De Neufville, 1975) have been important for successful institutionalization of social indicators throughout the
federal government:

- the agencies that collect and manipulate the data should be respected
and not subject to immediate political control,
- long-term financing and regular production of measures can be depended upon,
- the data are presented in a nonpolitical context,
- processes are established and followed for orderly changes in concepts and methods, and
- institutional arrangements exist to use and analyze the measure in
connection with policies.

In applying these criteria the Secretary will need to decide whether to
use an existing unit or create a new organization. An existing unit has the
advantages of a track record and experience in garnering support. The
disadvantage is that the monitoring function would compete with established functions for resources and attention.

The committee believes that the appropriate locus of responsibility for
the access monitoring activity is the federal government. Nevertheless, it
recognizes the important role that private foundations can play in stimulating government action and funding research and demonstration activities.

Racial and Ethnic Differences

Anyone reading this report will be struck by the persistent and in some
cases widening disparities between access to health care for blacks and
access for whites. Studies of health care access that compare the experience of whites with that of racial and ethnic minorities other than blacks
frequently reveal similar disparities. When certain factors, such as insurance status and income, are taken into account, some of the disparities
diminish. However, there is a continuing need to oversample minorities in
national surveys as well as to conduct specialized surveys focused on them.

Recommendation. Because it is not always feasible to improve the
accuracy of national data bases in recording the race or ethnicity of patients, it will be necessary to mount studies that better reveal the nature of
unexplained access problems for minorities.

FUTURE STEPS

The following lists present specific recommendations of the committee by indicator, together with the groups (e.g., researchers) or bodies (e.g., Public Health Service) to which the recommendation most pertains.

Objective 1: Promoting Successful Births

Indicator: Prenatal Care

1. Additional research (using revised birth records, among other sources) is needed to determine the relationships among medical risk factors, the content of prenatal care, and birth outcomes. (Researchers)

2. The National Center for Health Statistics should expedite the analysis and release of data from the 1988 National Maternal and Infant Health Survey and the 1990 longitudinal follow-up study. In addition to the potential value of these data in clarifying a range of issues related to the use of health care by pregnant women and infants, they should also be used to validate the accuracy of birth records. (National Center for Health Statistics, Public Health Service, States)

3. The National Center for Health Statistics and the states should consider including income and insurance data or, as an alternative, some indicator of poverty status on birth certificates. (Public Health Service, National Center for Health Statistics, States)

4. Efforts should continue to reach agreement on what constitutes adequate prenatal care and how to measure its provision. (Localities, Public Health Service, Researchers, States)

5. There is a need to enhance the capacity to conduct research on access barriers, such as lack of or inadequate insurance and low income, and their effects on the use of prenatal care. To this end, the development of automated birth and death records, to facilitate small-area analysis of data, would be helpful. (Localities, Researchers, States)

Indicator: Infant Mortality

1. Until income and insurance data are available on birth and death records, efforts should continue to link zip code information on birth records to census income data. (Researchers)

2. Research on how to measure infant mortality in ways that are sensitive to access should continue. The use of disease-specific death rates is one avenue that should be explored. (Researchers)

3. Research should continue on the increasing disparity between black and white infant mortality, with particular focus on the effects of specific barriers. (Researchers)

4. Wherever possible, data on Hispanics should be collected and analyzed according to individual ethnic subgroups. (National Center for Health Statistics, Public Health Service, States)

Indicator: Low Birthweight

1. Research and data analysis should focus on the large and growing disparity between the incidence of low-birthweight and very-low-birthweight infants among blacks and the incidence among other groups. (Researchers)

2. Better data are needed on barriers to access, especially concerning maternal income and insurance status. In the interim it may be possible to use data from the National Maternal and Infant Health Survey or from states that have linked data from Medicaid and birth records. Efforts should also continue to link zip code information on birth records with census income data to allow small-area analyses. (National Center for Health Statistics, Public Health Service, Researchers)

3. The Public Health Service should investigate ways to overcome delays between the collection of data and analysis and dissemination of vital statistics and survey information. (Public Health Service)

4. Research should continue into the differences in birth outcomes between first- and subsequent-generation mothers to gain a better understanding of how culture affects health care. (Researchers)

Indicator: Congenital Syphilis

1. To identify the root causes of congenital syphilis, additional research is necessary to investigate how access problems contribute to the large disparities between the incidence of primary and secondary syphilis for whites and that for blacks. (Researchers)

2. Further research is needed into the relationships among drug use, prenatal care, and congenital syphilis. The results of this research may allow interventions to be tailored to those afflicted by these complex social and health problems. (Researchers)

Objective 2: Reducing the Incidence of Vaccine-Preventable Childhood Diseases

Indicator: Preschool Immunization

1. The federal government should sponsor a school-based immunization reporting system under which schools would report to state health departments when entering students had completed their immunization schedules. The data would be aggregated at the federal level to provide a retrospective

picture of the proportion of preschool children who are routinely immunized. (Centers for Disease Control, Public Health Service)

2. Periodic supplements to the National Health Interview Survey on the topic of preschool immunization status should be continued, pending implementation of a school-based reporting system. (Centers for Disease Control, Public Health Service)

Indicator: Incidence of Vaccine-Preventable Childhood Diseases

1. Hospital admissions data and disease surveillance activities should be used more extensively to monitor outbreaks of infectious diseases. (Centers for Disease Control, Public Health Service, Researchers)

2. Surveillance activities of the Centers for Disease Control should be strengthened, and efforts to encourage local reporting should be increased. (Centers for Disease Control, Public Health Service)

3. Efforts to achieve more uniform and more complete reporting of infectious diseases, particularly among minorities, should be continued. (Centers for Disease Control, Public Health Service, States)

4. Research on the relationships among race, barriers to access, and infectious diseases should be encouraged. (Researchers)

Objective 3: Early Detection and Diagnosis
of Treatable Diseases

Indicator: Breast and Cervical Cancer Screening Procedures

1. Surveys of screening services should explore in depth why women do not seek screening. In particular, the surveys should assess the importance of access barriers, such as cost and lack of insurance coverage, to suboptimal use of screening. (Researchers)

2. The Behavioral Risk Factor Surveillance Survey should include questions on income, insurance status, and regular source of care. The results of these surveys can be relied upon for analysis when data from prevention or cancer supplements to the National Health Information Survey are not available. (Centers for Disease Control, Public Health Service)

Indicator: Incidence of Late-Stage Breast and Cervical Cancers

1. States should be encouraged to include in their cancer registries more information on a patient's socioeconomic and insurance status so that the effects of these barriers on access to care can be analyzed. When these data have been collected, they should be incorporated into the Surveillance, Epidemiology, and End Result (SEER) program of the National Cancer Insti-

tute. A clearinghouse is needed to compile data from all of the nation's tumor registries. (National Cancer Institute, Public Health Service)

2. In the interim, zip code information from birth certificates and census data on income should be linked to assess the importance of income as an access barrier. (Researchers)

3. Research is needed to determine why improvements in the rates of cancer screening among blacks are not reflected in improvements in early diagnosis, mortality rates, and survival compared with rates for whites. (Researchers)

Objective 4: Reducing the Effects of Chronic Diseases and Prolonging Life

Indicator: Continuing Care for Chronic Diseases

1. A longitudinal survey of individuals with chronic diseases should be conducted. (National Center for Health Statistics)

2. In the interim the National Health Interview Survey should incorporate questions about access either in its disease-specific supplements or in the core portion of the survey. (National Center for Health Statistics, Public Health Service)

Indicator: High-Cost Discretionary Care

1. The reasons some groups fail to use discretionary medical procedures need further attention. Resource barriers, patient and physician attitudes, and over- and underutilization of services need to be taken into account, along with financial barriers, if this indicator is to be correctly interpreted. (Health Care Financing Administration, Researchers)

2. Additional referral-sensitive procedures should be explored to determine whether they might be added to the basic list. (Researchers)

Indicator: Avoidable Hospitalization for Chronic Diseases

1. All states should require hospitals to maintain discharge data bases.

2. States should explore the feasibility of incorporating income data and information to help determine severity of illness on the hospital discharge record. (Researchers)

3. Studies are needed on the dynamics of patient care-seeking behavior. These studies should focus on ambulatory-care-sensitive conditions and physician admitting practices. The results of such research would be useful for interpreting differences in admission rates among groups and the relative contributions of various access barriers to delayed or poor-quality care. (Researchers)

Indicator: Access-Related Excess Mortality

1. The committee has demonstrated the potential of applying risk adjustments to mortality data to better understand the contribution of access problems to premature mortality. Further work is needed to develop models that can produce a more refined measure of access-related mortality. In addition, these models should be used to consider not only blacks but also other relevant population groups, such as other racial/ethnic groups and low-income populations. (Centers for Disease Control, Researchers)

2. Improved models will require better and more up-to-date data on the mortality risks of various populations. In addition to continued epidemiological follow-up surveys, there is a need to determine whether useful information could be extracted from routine surveys, such as the National Health Interview Survey. (National Center for Health Statistics)

Objective 5: Reducing Morbidity and Pain Through Timely and Appropriate Treatment

Indicator: Acute Medical Care

1. The National Center for Health Statistics should explore methods that can be used to improve our understanding of what constitutes timely and appropriate use of physician services during episodes of acute illness.

Indicator: Dental Services

1. The National Health Interview Survey's supplements on dental services should gather more detailed information about income- and insurance-related barriers to care. The surveys should also distinguish more fully among the broad classes of procedures performed. (National Center for Health Statistics)

Indicator: Avoidable Hospitalization for Acute Conditions

1. Research should focus on factors that lead to the hospitalization of people with acute diseases. Surveys of patients and admitting physicians, both in the emergency room and in inpatient settings, are needed. (Researchers)

REFERENCE

De Neufville, J. I. 1975. *Social Indicators and Public Policy.* New York: Elsevier.

APPENDIXES

A

Developing Indicators of Access to Care: The Case for HIV Disease

Vincent Mor [1]

Since the first case was diagnosed in 1981, acquired immune deficiency syndrome, or AIDS, has become a leading cause of death among men age 25 to 44; more than 100,000 persons died of AIDS in 1981-1990 (CDC, 1990). The most recent Centers for Disease Control (CDC) projections are that as many as 153,000 persons were living with AIDS at the end of 1991 and that approximately 1 million persons are infected with the human immunodeficiency virus (HIV; CDC, 1991). Cumulatively, 275,000 cases of AIDS will have been reported by the end of 1991. Initially, the concentration of AIDS cases was in a few urban areas on the East and West coasts, but the incidence rate has been rising in communities outside the original epicenters, more rapidly in some risk groups than in the first-line cities.

The epidemic was first associated with homosexual contact, but HIV transmission through injection drug practice has been increasing in urban centers all along the East coast and even in the rural South. Linked to, but independent of, the rise in drug-related transmission is the incidence of AIDS among women and their children, which is expected to increase by about one-third per year. The incidence rate among bisexual and homosexual males in New York City, San Francisco, and Los Angeles who do not use drugs has actually been flat over the past several years. (Incidence is rising in this group in other areas of the country, however.) Given these

[1] Vincent Mor is Director and Associate Professor of Medical Science at the Center for Gerontology and Health Care Research, Brown University, Providence, Rhode Island.

changing rates, the concentration of this epidemic will continue to increase in the nation's poor, drug-using, and minority populations.

The availability of effective curative and prophylactic treatments such as zidovudine (AZT) and pentamadine has provided a clinical rationale for early diagnosis (Fischl et al., 1987; Volberding et al., 1990). Life expectancy for those diagnosed with AIDS has been increasing over the first decade of the epidemic, even controlling for the changing pattern of diagnosed diseases that constitute the case definition of AIDS (CDC, 1990; Harris, 1990; Lemp et al., 1990; Piette et al., in press). Earlier diagnosis, longer survival, and extended years of medical treatment all imply that AIDS has become a chronic disease requiring a complex mix of health and social services that must be modulated as a patient's disease status and treatment affect both physiological and social functioning (Benjamin, 1988; Mechanic and Aiken, 1989).

Since the early days of the epidemic, the technology for treating and managing the multiplicity of opportunistic infections in AIDS has changed rapidly (Cohen et al., 1990). Variation in the length of hospital stays has also been repeatedly noted by region and provider (Andrulis et al., 1989; Kaplowitz et al., 1988; Seage et al., 1990). Recent studies have shown that experience with AIDS management has a positive impact on survival and that more experienced facilities appear to make more effective use of additional resources, compared with those with less experience (Bennett et al., 1990). Accompanying the change in clinical practice has been a reduction in the duration of hospital stays (Seage et al., 1990) and an increase in the use of outpatient and home treatment with "high-tech" nursing care (e.g., home intravenous units, infusion and parenteral nutrition).

Because of both the rapid impoverishment of formerly employed persons who lose their private health insurance and the increasing prevalence of AIDS among the previously poor and uninsured, urban municipal and not-for-profit hospitals are disproportionately paying the price of the AIDS epidemic (Andrulis, 1989; Baily et al., 1990; Green and Arno, 1990). Since many of these institutions are facing other pressures, such as homelessness and the medical consequences of drug abuse, the unique pressures of AIDS only serve to complicate their ability to address an already complex mix of social problems.

Public reaction to the AIDS epidemic has been volatile and generally negative (Blendon and Donelan, 1988). Each new incident of transmission that breaks prior stereotypes is greeted with fear and hysteria in certain sectors. (The recent case of HIV transmission from a dentist to his patients provides a graphic example of this phenomenon.) At the same time, a substantial minority blame the victims for the behavioral transgressions that "caused" their condition (Blendon and Donelan, 1988). This prejudice isolates infected individuals and leads to job discrimination, denial of insurance benefits, and reduced access to personal health care.

With this background, HIV disease can serve as a sensitive indicator of the degree of access to personal health care services in the United States. However, relatively little is known about the reduced access experienced by this population, how to measure it, or what it means. Further conceptualization of these issues is required before specific indicators of reduced access can be suggested with any confidence.

Following the model proposed by the IOM Committee for Monitoring Access to Personal Health Services in Chapter 2, this paper reviews the issues and existing knowledge about the presence of barriers to access to health services that confront persons with HIV disease. The consequences for persons with HIV disease are also examined by measuring variations in utilization of health services. This review relies not only on the relatively sparse published literature but also on quantitative data and qualitative insights derived from an ongoing study examining the organization and delivery of health and social services to persons with AIDS in various cities around the country. This study is described briefly below, after which the relevant literature is reviewed and new data on these issues are presented. The last section of this paper proposes a series of indicators of barriers to access and the types of data systems necessary to monitor them.

ROBERT WOOD JOHNSON FOUNDATION AIDS HEALTH SERVICES PROGRAM AND EVALUATION

Between 1986 and 1990 the Robert Wood Johnson Foundation (RWJF) funded nine projects (AIDS Health Services Programs [AHSP]) in 11 cities to develop and coordinate specialized health and supportive community services for persons with disabling HIV disease (Mor et al., 1989). The emphasis in these projects was on developing networks of community-based care providers to offer new services and to coordinate the delivery of existing services. The central organizational features of the programs were a formal consortium of participating agencies and individualized case management. Program evaluation was conducted by Brown University's Center for Gerontology and Health Care Research, under the direction of this author. The evaluation integrates quantitative data obtained from computerized program "intake" records and two longitudinal cohorts of program clients. Clients were surveyed about their experience in obtaining health services and qualitative information was obtained from four rounds of site visits and a detailed review of program progress reports, correspondence, and budgets.

Several papers based on this evaluation have already appeared or are in press (Capilouto et al., 1991; Fleishman, 1990; Fleishman et al., 1989, 1990, 1991; Mor et al., 1989, 1992; Piette et al., 1990, in press; Stein et al., 1991). The major evaluation issues pertaining to the success of consortia building and case management as vehicles for service integration are still being examined. The project information presented in succeeding sections represents both published and unpublished data. The more qualitative information is based largely on case studies; the quantitative information clearly is limited by its focus on program clients rather than on the experience of a broad cross section of persons with HIV disease in each city. Nonetheless, because this data source contains specific, detailed information relevant to the access barriers that confront those with HIV disease, it is useful as an illustrative device.

ISSUES IN ASSESSING ACCESS TO PERSONAL HEALTH CARE

Equitable access to health care services has been a major focus of health services research in the United States for four decades (Ginzberg, 1990). Research in the past two decades has emphasized factors associated with the rising costs of health care; now, as a result of growth in the number of uninsured over the past decade, access to care has once again emerged as a central topic in health services research. This section reviews the various barriers to use of services confronting persons with HIV disease. In keeping with the model proposed by the IOM committee, barriers have been classified as financial, structural, personal, and attitudinal. Each is defined in relation to the special issues facing persons with HIV disease.

Financial Barriers

Financial barriers to access to health care services include insurance coverage, provider reimbursement rates, and lack of investment in resources designated for the treatment of HIV disease. Other financial barriers can also be noted, such as out-of-pocket expenses for patients, the high cost of treatment, and the substantial indirect costs of the disease to the patient and society. These barriers are either covered under one of the topics mentioned above or are beyond the scope of this paper.

Insurance Coverage

The absence of insurance coverage is a barrier to health care services regardless of a person's medical problems. In the case of HIV disease, however, the poverty and/or limited work history and savings of the population at risk, as well as the increasingly prolonged nature of the disease, mean that those infected are likely to endure limited access over a long period of time. Because the absence of private compared with public insurance may have a different, and potentially sequential, impact on the person with HIV disease, these two issues are treated separately.

Private insurance is almost always tied to employment, because the purchase of individual health insurance coverage is quite expensive and replete with coverage restrictions (Eby, 1989). Loss of employment traditionally has signaled loss of insurance. With passage of the Comprehensive Omnibus Budget Reconciliation Act of 1988, however, individuals have the right to continue purchasing health insurance from their previous employer, paying all the premiums themselves, for up to 18 months. Anecdotal evidence from many sources suggests that the loss of employment income, ongoing living expenses, and increased out-of-pocket medical expenses for copayments make paying these insurance premiums impractical, even at the group rate. The recent Ryan White bill (P.L. 101-381) allows states to pay these premiums. No data are available to estimate the proportion of formerly employed persons with HIV disease who are paying their own health insurance premiums.

There is also a dearth of data by which to quantify the rate at which loss of private insurance occurs following either onset of symptoms or formal AIDS diagnosis. Yelin and his colleagues (1991) report on the time between initial HIV symptom onset and work cessation in a cohort of 170 patients treated at San Francisco General Hospital. Three years after initial symptoms appeared, less than half of these patients were working; another 12 percent had reduced work loads.

Martin and colleagues surveyed 432 HIV-positive persons in Texas in 1988 (40 percent of distributed questionnaires were returned). The proportion of respondents with private insurance was only 41 percent (Martin et al., 1989). Kass (1989), comparing participants in the Multicenter AIDS Cohort Studies (MACS) with leukemia patients, reported that people with AIDS were more likely to be uninsured and more likely to have been turned down for insurance.

Based on intake records completed for all clients of the RWJF AHSPs, only 21.3 percent of some 14,000 clients were employed full-time at their entry into the program, and only half of these had private insurance. This result is consistent with the finding that many of the uninsured in the United States are employed. Half of those who were unemployed when they entered the program had no health insurance at all, either private or public.

Although it is likely that only a minority of all individuals with significant symptomatic HIV disease have private medical insurance, the impact of AIDS on specific private insurers is not insignificant. MetLife reviewed health claims for 1986–1989. In 1989, 6,450 people received group medical claim payments for AIDS-related diseases for a total of $111.2 million (Pickett et al., 1990). This figure constitutes almost a 300 percent increase over the AIDS-related claims incurred by the company in 1986.

Little evidence exists about how the insurance coverage of persons with HIV changes with disease progression. Kaufman and his colleagues

(1990) linked hospital discharge records in the state of New York between 1984 and 1986 and found that 17 percent of the patients whose status on first admission was as a private payer had been changed to government reimbursement by their last indicated admission. Unfortunately, the authors do not note the proportion of patients who had no insurance coverage at all. The Texas sample surveyed by Martin and colleagues reported that 60 percent were privately insured at initial HIV diagnosis and 41 percent were insured at the time of the survey (Martin et al., 1989). Interviews with a nonrandomized sample of 1,386 program clients in 9 of the 11 cities funded by the RWJF revealed that 44 percent reported having had private insurance at the time that they learned they had HIV disease. Of those, 37 percent had lost their insurance within three to six months.

Access to personal health care services appears to be strongly linked to the availability of private insurance coverage. Zucconi and her colleagues surveyed HIV-positive men and found that the number of reported physician visits was strongly associated with being insured (Zucconi et al., 1989). Those RWJF survey sample clients with private insurance reported significantly more physician and clinic visits than those without insurance and were significantly less likely to use an emergency room (Mor et al., 1992). However, in neither that study nor one by Seage and colleagues (1990) was there a relationship between having private insurance and the probability of being hospitalized.

Although loss of insurance may be the longitudinal experience of individuals, changes in the insurance mix of the HIV population will occur as the composition of the population shifts and as early identification and treatment of HIV disease become more commonplace. The growth of public insurance coverage for medical treatment of HIV disease undoubtedly will increase with the changing population (Green and Arno, 1990); in addition, the liability of private insurers may grow to cover the early treatment expenses of those with HIV disease who are still employed. Given the promise of early intervention efforts among those with asymptomatic HIV disease, this is an issue of importance for the near future (Arno et al., 1990). Considerable concern has been voiced about the private insurance industry's willingness to continue to provide coverage to persons with high-cost conditions such as HIV (Lipson, 1988; Parmet, 1987); however, the empirical documentation of instances of coverage rejection, withdrawals, and limitations is difficult. Kass (1989) reported that 11 percent of AIDS cases had been turned down for health insurance. As one part of the RWJF program evaluation, 355 clients in three cities were asked about their experience with private insurance. Of those who had health insurance at the time of HIV diagnosis, 40 percent subsequently lost it. For most (23 out of 54 persons), this occurred because they were no longer employed; the rest lost their coverage because their policy was terminated or they were no longer able to pay the premiums.

Denial of coverage on the basis of retrospective interpretations of pre-HIV diagnosis claims and the widespread adoption of HIV testing as a precondition for health and life insurance applications are strategies being used by the insurance industry to limit liability (IOM, 1986). Indeed, a 1987 survey of state laws revealed that only eight states forbid HIV testing by insurers (Faden and Kass, 1988). Moreover, the growing cost of health insurance premiums for employers may make companies increasingly willing to adopt "carve-out" and prior-condition exemption practices to limit the perceived catastrophic effect of high-cost AIDS patients in their group.

Public insurance is playing an ever-increasing role as a payer for health and social services for persons with AIDS (Green and Arno, 1990). Between 1983 and 1987 in New York City, Los Angeles, and San Francisco, the percentage of hospitalizations of AIDS patients financed by Medicaid increased between 50 percent and 100 percent, whereas the percentage financed by private insurance dropped between 25 percent and 50 percent. When compared with non-AIDS cases, costs for AIDS admissions were 50 percent to 275 percent more likely to have been paid by Medicaid than by private insurance. According to the U.S. AIDS Hospital Survey (Andrulis et al., 1989), there is considerable regional variation in the payer source mix for hospitalizations. In 1987, among public hospitals in the East, 71 percent of admissions were paid by Medicaid; it paid for only 18 percent of admissions to public hospitals in the South. Private hospitals are also less likely to serve Medicaid patients in all regions but the South. In contrast, nearly half of all outpatient visits by AIDS patients to private hospitals were covered by Medicaid in virtually all regions. Public hospitals, particularly in the South and West, were much more likely than private hospitals to incur "bad debt" or to use local financing to offer free outpatient clinic care to AIDS patients.

Green and Arno (1990) found that in Los Angeles, almost all (98.9 percent) privately insured AIDS admissions occurred in private hospitals, whereas only 42 percent of Medicaid admissions went to private hospitals. Similar patterns were observed in the other cities studied. The authors remark that "the differences are so large . . . as to suggest nearly distinct systems of care depending upon type of insurance." Site visit experience in the 11 RWJF AHSP demonstration communities reinforced this notion of a bifurcated system.

Regional variation in reliance on Medicaid is due to the enormous variation among the states in eligibility policies. Unless a state has a categorical eligibility program (e.g., Aid to Families with Dependent Children, or AFDC) or a program for the medically needy, individuals must meet state income and asset tests before they are eligible to receive Medicaid. And even the presence of a medically needy program does not guarantee continuous coverage under Medicaid in most states. The income test in some is below 50 percent of the poverty line, meaning that individuals who have become presumptively eligible for Social Security Disability Income (SSDI) may receive just enough money to make them ineligible for Medicaid. States like Texas and Louisiana have very low income limits for Medicaid.

The services covered under Medicaid also vary considerably by state. Some, like Louisiana, arbitrarily limit the number of inpatient care days as well as the number of physician and home health visits covered by Medicaid. Almost all Medicaid programs have updated their pharmacy formulary to include treatment drugs such as AZT and pentamadine (Buchanan, 1988), although in some states there is a perception of limited public supply.

Some states have chosen to expand the range of services that can be provided to Medicaid recipients (e.g., home care, case management, homemaker, transportation, and home medical visits) by requesting "waivers" from the Health Care Financing Administration (HCFA). HCFA approval of a waiver depends on a state's demonstration of how the waiver will produce savings. Expanding home services as a substitute for more expensive inpatient care is almost always the rationale. This means that publicly insured persons with AIDS in waivered states will have access to a broader, more diverse array of health care services than will be the case for all but the most fortunate patients with private insurance. New Jersey has had waivers in place since 1987; other states, however, have such limited Medicaid coverage that it is virtually impossible to demonstrate how the waivers would be cost neutral, much less produce savings. Even when a case can be made for cost savings, when properly evaluated these programs almost always result in higher costs.

The time lapse between loss of private coverage and eligibility for public insurance may be prolonged. The devastating personal effects of this lapse may result in impoverishment, since home ownership (the one asset spared by Medicaid spend-down rules) is not the norm in this population. (Only 10.8 percent of respondents to the RWJF survey owned their own homes.) In examining respondent satisfaction with the health care they received, the RWJF survey found that those who previously had private insurance but were no longer covered reported significantly lower satisfaction with their access to health care. During the interim, from the time people lose their private insurance to the time they become eligible for public coverage, there is some evidence that outpatient and physician visits are less frequent (Mor et al., 1989; Zucconi et al., 1989). If these individuals require hospitalization, the hospitals that accept them (presumably public facilities) incur added bad debt.

Provider Reimbursement Rates

Provider reimbursement levels also may affect access to the personal health care system. It is well documented that patients with Medicaid as their primary source of payment for health care have a more difficult time finding a private physician to treat them (Holahan, 1984; Perloff et al., 1987). A major reason is that Medicaid reimbursement rates tend to be substantially lower than customary charges and reimbursements from other payers. If a provider receives lower-than-average levels of reimbursement for treating Medicaid patients and AIDS patients cost more to treat than the average patient, the provider may be even more reluctant to treat AIDS patients. The implications of inadequate reimbursement for the AIDS patient may differ for hospitals, clinics, physicians, home health providers, and nursing homes. Consequently, they are discussed separately below.

The cost-to-charge ratios of hospitals reflect whether, for various types of services, their accounting cost for producing a service is higher or lower than what they charge for it. This cost in turn might differ from their reimbursement for the service by third-party payers. Andrulis and his colleagues (1989) surveyed U.S. hospitals and asked them to estimate their costs per inpatient day and per outpatient visit for treating AIDS patients. Across all regions, both public and private hospitals reported losing from $4 per patient day among private hospitals in the South to $386 per day among southern public hospitals. Reporting hospitals also noted that they were experiencing losses with non-AIDS medical/surgical patients, but these losses were substantially lower. Similar findings were reported for outpatient visits.

Hospitals that note discrepancies between costs incurred and reimbursements received for AIDS hospital admissions may attempt to minimize their exposure to financial risk by limiting the number of AIDS admissions, particularly those insured by Medicaid. Green and Arno (1990), as well as Andrulis and coworkers (1987a), have shown that Medicaid patients are underrepresented among AIDS admissions to private hospitals, compared with public hospitals.

The hospital outpatient clinic has become a central point of treatment for persons with HIV disease. Public hospitals have a long tradition of providing care to the poor and uninsured, and these clinics are training sites for medical schools and affiliated academic medical centers. Andrulis and colleagues (1987a) found an average of 161 HIV outpatients (median = 36) with an average of 1,460 visits per year in the 80 public hospitals they surveyed. On average, the 196 private hospitals surveyed served far fewer outpatients. Whether this differential is due to the diversion of high-cost, low-reimbursement patients to the public sector or to the fact that few private hospitals specialize in this care is not known at this time.

Access to physician services can also be compromised by the rate at which physicians are reimbursed relative to their "cost" for providing a particular service. Green and Arno (1990) revealed that in both New York City and San Francisco, Medicaid pays between 10 and 50 percent of what private insurance companies reimburse for the same service. For example, in New York, Medicaid pays only $11 for an office visit with a new patient, whereas a private insurer pays $84. In San Francisco, chemotherapy with infusion is reimbursed at $12 by Medicaid and at $28 by a private insurance carrier.

Conversations with medical personnel held during visits to the RWJF cities to educate the medical community about HIV treatment techniques revealed that, in many localities, only a small cadre of physicians care for persons with HIV disease. Rizzo and his colleagues analyzed responses of the 1988 American Medical Association (AMA) physician survey and found that about one-half of all physicians reported having treated at least one HIV-positive person (Rizzo et al., 1990). Although there is no hard evidence, many physicians who are willing to treat patients with HIV disease transfer them to the care of the public hospital clinic once a patient's private insurance lapses. They indicate that they do not treat patients without insurance and, given the low reimbursement rates, will retain ongoing continuity of care responsibility for only a small number of patients who become covered by Medicaid.

Nursing homes have not played a prominent role in meeting the health and social service needs of AIDS patients in most communities in the United States. Only 4 of 47 skilled nursing facilities surveyed in Oregon in 1989 had served an AIDS patient (White and Berger, 1991). Marder and Linsk (1990) documented that none of 42 hospitalized persons with AIDS who required discharge arrangements were placed in a nursing home. Similar experiences have been reported by hospital discharge planners and case managers in the cities funded by the RWJF. With certain exceptions (e.g., publicly operated county facilities), the nursing home industry has not served persons with HIV disease.

Although there are many reasons for this phenomenon, one that is frequently mentioned is inadequate reimbursement. Recently, several states have instituted "enriched" Medicaid reimbursement for AIDS patients in nursing facilities. For example, Florida providers receive a supplemental fee of nearly $75 per diem for serving AIDS patients—almost double what the state pays for a patient without AIDS. Nonetheless, as recently as the winter of 1991, only one nongovernmental facility in south Florida admitted persons with AIDS. Providers in locations as disparate as Minnesota, Florida, and California all maintain that it costs $200 a day to care for an AIDS patient in a nursing home, and in California no supplement is available. Swan and his colleagues, reporting the results of a time and motion study of

93 persons with AIDS in California nursing homes, found that they required 6.5 hours of nursing time per day, which is a much higher rate than that for traditional nursing home patients (Swan et al., 1990). Providers say that the specialized reimbursement is still inadequate.

New York is developing AIDS residential health care facilities (RHCF) to provide subacute care, rehabilitative care, active nursing treatment, palliative care, and case management services. The state has approved more than 200 beds, and some facilities have been established in New York City and Rochester. These facilities, as well as specialized AIDS health-related facilities (HRF) or nursing homes, are to be paid a substantially higher rate than facilities serving other nursing home patients, both because they entail a new class of licensed facility and to encourage providers to offer this service for AIDS patients. Presumably, this effort will reduce the access barriers facing those with advanced HIV disease in New York.

In view of the major emphasis on community-based care for persons with HIV disease, the role of home health agencies (HHA) is critical. The recent study in Oregon by White and Berger (1991) found that 13 of 16 agencies located in areas with a relatively high prevalence of HIV had served persons with AIDS. Fleishman and Masterson-Allen (1991) surveyed 263 HHAs in 11 cities with high rates of HIV infection and found that 76 percent of these agencies had served patients with HIV, although only 57 percent had served an AIDS patient in the past three months. Smaller, proprietary agencies and those without Medicaid certification were less likely than other agencies to have ever served an HIV-infected patient. However, in areas with many HHAs, it appears that a higher proportion of agencies able to provide intensive home nursing are willing and anxious to do so.

HHAs noted that reimbursement was a major barrier to serving AIDS patients (Fleishman and Masterson-Allen, 1991). A study by the Home Care Association of New York determined that AIDS patients "need 13 percent more nursing time than terminal cancer patients and 29 percent more than the average home care patient" (DeHovitz, 1990). Based on this study, the average nursing visit rate for HIV-infected patients in New York was increased by 30 percent in 1988.

An obvious barrier to receiving home care or home hospice benefits is the lack of housing. Numerous studies have documented the difficulty of discharging AIDS patients from the hospital because of a lack of housing alternatives. Fleishman and Masterson-Allen (1991) also found that home health agencies reported that the greatest difficulty associated with serving AIDS patients was the absence of a stable home environment. According to their respondents, this problem was compounded by the fact that in many communities those with HIV disease lived in the least safe neighborhoods, thereby requiring personal guards or other costly strategies to ensure the safety of nurses and aides.

It is precisely this higher cost of caring for persons with AIDS that has made hospices anxious about assuming the liability for all medical care of persons with AIDS who elect to be served by a hospice. Since 1989, coverage of hospice services by Medicaid has been mandated in all states: hospices can now receive standard, prospectively set reimbursement for home and inpatient care. The hospice is responsible, however, for all medical services consumed including hospitalization, drugs, and infusion therapies. Because AIDS treatment standards are evolving rapidly, optimal strategies for symptom relief might require hospitalization or continuous infusion at home, or both; these services are extraordinarily costly even if persons with AIDS elect palliation and no aggressive care. It is little wonder that hospices are ambivalent about enrolling patients with AIDS as hospice beneficiaries and, depending on state reimbursement levels, may choose to provide similar care as an HHA rather than a hospice (personal communications to the author during site visits in Florida and Louisiana).

Investment in Resources for Treating HIV Disease

Investment in treatment resources by the state, county, or local municipality has clearly had an effect on access to personal health care for persons with HIV disease across the country. Rowe and Ryan (1988) catalogued state expenditures for AIDS between 1986 and 1988. Florida, California, New York, and New Jersey were among the highest spenders. Direct expenditures for patient care climbed from 4 percent to 19 percent of the total between 1986 and 1988, largely because of the added emphasis on direct care in New York. In general, however, most of the state expenditures were directed toward education, testing, and counseling.

The most obvious examples of local investment are the public-sector hospitals. Some have their own tax base in the county or metropolitan area property tax. The budgets of others may derive from direct line-item allocations by the state legislature. In Louisiana, for example, Charity Hospital in New Orleans was designated a statewide referral center for AIDS treatment, education, and training. In this particular instance, given Louisiana's limited Medicaid program, the concentrated state investment in the Charity Hospital AIDS program has enhanced access to high-quality outpatient care far beyond what would have been possible if the hospital were relying only on Medicaid reimbursement.

Another example is the transformation in West Palm Beach County of hospital districts with their own taxing authorities into a countywide "health district" with spending authority to cover not only hospital care but home and community care as well. Although the referendum covered all aspects of health care for the poor and uninsured (there are no public hospitals in the county), the first beneficiaries were the many uninsured patients with

HIV disease and the public clinics and programs serving that population. Providers benefit from guaranteed funding of AIDS patients care, and patients benefit from increased access and choice.

Structural Barriers

Structural barriers to access to the personal health care system have traditionally included lack of a primary source of care, lack of appropriate service providers in one's area, distance from providers, and extended waiting time for providers. In each case, these structural barriers theoretically detract from the patient's ability and willingness to obtain, and then adhere to, appropriate medical care.

Lack of a Primary Source of Care

Having a regular source of ambulatory care has traditionally been viewed as a sine qua non for access to medical care. Without a regular source of care, it is argued, individuals will not have the benefits of preventive care and periodic checkups. When they do become ill, there will be no one who is sufficiently knowledgeable to make informed clinical decisions about their treatment. National surveys have consistently shown that the 15 percent of the population without a regular source of care are less likely to be insured and to have had recommended screening exams (Hayward et al., 1991).

Although in the general population the proportion of people without a regular source of care is only 15 percent, this figure may be higher among those with HIV disease. In the general population, the groups most likely not to have a regular source of care, men between 18 and 45 and those without insurance, are precisely the groups with HIV disease. An added difficulty in trying to estimate the proportion of HIV-infected people without regular care is the lack of comparability between populations. Because HIV disproportionately strikes those who are underrepresented in national telephone surveys (the method used to ascertain those with a regular source of care), it is improper to extrapolate these national estimates to the HIV population.

Several major issues complicate an understanding of what is and is not a "usual source of care" for persons with HIV disease: (1) the nature of the relationship between nonmedical treatment systems and medical care providers; (2) the role of the hospital clinic and whether, with its rotating staff, it provides the continuity generally associated with a primary care physician; (3) the role of disease progression in stimulating a shift in primary care responsibility from the generalist to the specialist; and (4) the implications of using multiple physicians in the ongoing care of a patient.

Persons with HIV disease who are active intravenous drug abusers form the group that is least likely to have a usual source of care (Mor et al., 1992). This finding raises concerns about how the drug treatment and medical care systems interact. The impact of drug use on the health care system has been well documented and appears to be growing, particularly in New York (Myers et al., 1990). The number of drug- and alcohol-related hospital discharges throughout the state increased 1 percent per year. In New York City, discharges, patient days, and length of stay for those with substance abuse diagnoses have been increasing at rates of more than 10 percent a year. In 1987, in New York City, "one out of every seven patient days for AIDS care was devoted to patients with both AIDS and substance abuse diagnoses" (Myers et al., 1990) and it is this group of individuals with dual diagnoses that is increasing most rapidly.

Little information is available to indicate where these individuals obtain ambulatory medical care, although many observers believe that they rely on hospital emergency rooms. Drug treatment programs, whether residential or outpatient (and with or without methadone maintenance) have tended not to be connected to medical treatment systems, despite the high risk of medical complications associated with illicit drug use. The state of New York has begun to recognize this failing, given the growing HIV sero-prevalence rate among intravenous drug users, and has instituted various demonstration projects to open "multi-modality treatment centers which would include outpatient, inpatient, enhanced methadone services, AIDS services, central intake," and other services, all provided in one setting. In addition, the existing substance abuse network is being linked to primary health and mental health services. Whether this approach will reduce the rate of hospitalizations that occur through the emergency room among Medicaid-funded, HIV-infected persons in New York City remains to be seen.

The hospital clinic is often the only option available for persons with AIDS. (However, few data are available concerning the relative proportion of persons with HIV disease served by hospital clinics, compared with private physicians' offices.) Among 408 respondents to the RWJF AHSP evaluation who were clients of a community-based social service agency, only 38 percent reported that their usual source of care was a private physician or health maintenance organizations, whereas 44 percent named the clinic at the local public hospital. Among those identified in the RWJF public hospital clinic sample, almost all (95 percent) named the clinic as their usual source of care.

The public hospital clinics in RWJF communities have evolved from being merely infectious disease specialty clinics into continuity of care clinics. In some, a concerted effort is made to establish primary care teams that follow a panel of patients. Often, these clinics are staffed by the most experienced physicians treating HIV in that community, a strong incentive to receive care there even among those individuals who have private health insurance.

Based on site visits to and telephone contact with clinics in non-RWJF cities, it appears that the transformation of traditional public hospital medical clinics into primary care programs has occurred in other cities as well. The clinic environment remains complex, since many patients are followed by special research clinics that may or may not involve the same medical staff as in the regular clinic. Yet this problem of a multiplicity of providers complicated by participation in research protocols is not unique to the public clinic patient population. Indeed, being treated in multiple care settings may be more burdensome for the private patient, particularly as this inevitably involves travel from one location to another and not just shifting from clinic to clinic in the hospital. Using a public hospital clinic rather than a private physician as a regular source of care does not necessarily signify poorer quality or less continuity.

These growing "islands of excellence" in the public hospital system will, however, come under increasing pressure with early identification of patients for prophylactic therapy. This swelling group, many of whom are uninsured, cannot reasonably be accommodated by the existing capacity of public hospital-based clinics. Staff in the RWJF study found that time spent by newly diagnosed, asymptomatic individuals on a waiting list in a community often is six months or longer. In some locations, health planners are making a concerted effort to arrange a system of linkages between publicly supported community health centers and the public hospital HIV specialty centers. In some areas, these locations are linked to existing sexually transmitted disease clinics; in other areas, HIV-infected individuals are integrated into community health centers.

Lack of Appropriate Service Providers

It is still unclear what pattern of patient transfer from generalist to specialist is most appropriate in the case of HIV disease. (This level of uncertainty is not surprising; there are few standards for this process for any chronic disease.) The process of referral and transfer is complicated by insurance coverage, negative attitudes toward HIV-infected patients, and the varied expertise of the physicians from many different backgrounds who specialize in AIDS care. It is possible that HIV disease may become a subspecialty within medicine. Indeed, there are already examples of divisions of HIV, separate from divisions of infectious disease, emerging within departments of medicine at major medical schools.

A related issue pertains to the implications for patients of receiving care from many different physicians. Theoretically, the rationale for a single, regular source of care is that this provider will be most knowledgeable about the patient's condition, values, and preferences. In the event that specialty care is required, the primary source of care should be able to coordinate it and to integrate the results of multiple consultations. Unfortunately, there is little empirical evidence to substantiate the success of this model for any chronic disease, much less HIV disease. Consequently, no data suggest that seeing several physicians is more or less appropriate than seeing one primary physician.

Data from the survey of RWJF AHSP participants whose regular source of care was the public hospital clinic revealed that 11 percent also saw a private physician and 9 percent reported a clinic visit to a different hospital. Among those with a private physician as their usual source of care, 16 percent reported also using the public hospital clinic. Across both groups of respondents, nearly 15 percent reported having used three or more different sources of care in the past four months, and only 43 percent reported using only one source. This pattern was no more likely for patients whose regular source of care was a public hospital clinic than it was for those whose usual source of care was a private physician.

Whether seeing multiple physicians in different locations actually leads to more diffuse care still needs to be investigated. Factors such as these will provide an interesting indicator of continuity of care, once the practice and its consequences are better understood.

Distance from Care Providers

The distance patients with HIV disease must travel to obtain medical care may influence compliance with recommended medical regimens. As long as the epidemic remained within the confines of urban centers and their suburban environs, distance or travel time was not a major impediment unless the patient was seriously impaired or homebound. For example, the survey of RWJF program clients found that 70 percent of respondents traveled less than 30 minutes to reach the clinic or their physician, and only 14 percent traveled more than 45 minutes. Nonetheless, even this relatively short travel time can present insurmountable problems for some patients. Although only 32 percent of RWJF survey clients needed assistance with transportation, for most of that group (70 percent) this need was unmet. In fact, the lack of assistance with transportation was greatest among the most physically impaired. Thus, even though transportation problems affect only a minority of patients, when present, they constitute a major barrier.

Extended Waiting Times for Providers

Waiting time in public hospital clinics is traditionally long and a principal complaint among patients. Perception of waiting time is strongly correlated with other measures of access to medical care such as satisfaction with access. Theoretically, perceptions about waiting time may affect compliance because patients may be more likely to miss scheduled appointments if they anticipate a long wait. The survey of RWJF program clients found that 35 percent routinely waited more than an hour for an appointment; only 36 percent reported routinely waiting less than half an hour. In response to the question, How would you rate your satisfaction with the length of time spent waiting?, more than 30 percent said "fair" or "poor," and another 30 percent said merely "good." Generally, responses to such questions on satisfaction are heavily weighted toward the positive. The strongly negative ratings on this aspect of access clearly indicate that waiting time is a problem.

Public clinics have long waiting lists, which means that individuals seeking medical care will be triaged unless their condition is serious. Site visit discussions with public HIV clinics in RWJF demonstration and non-demonstration communities revealed that waits of six months or longer were standard for asymptomatic HIV-infected individuals seeking treatment and a source of primary care knowledgeable about HIV disease. Such extended waits can be seen as a real deterrent to care and presumably are far more characteristic of the public than of the private health care system.

The availability of providers who care for persons with HIV disease is not well quantified. Anecdotal evidence from conversations with staff from public hospitals and community-based organizations suggests that in most communities, only a handful of physicians are willing to treat HIV patients.

In 1985, one-half of the physicians not specializing in radiology or pathology who responded to the AMA socioeconomic monitoring system survey reported that they had treated at least one HIV-positive patient. This finding, however, provides little basis for estimating the proportion of primary care physicians who retain clinical management responsibility for these patients, as has been recommended (Northfelt et al., 1988; Rizzo et al., 1990). Indeed, the call has been sounded from various quarters for general internists to assume primary care responsibility for persons with HIV disease by engaging in clinical tasks as diverse as sexual counseling to managing the administration of retroviral agents (American College of Physicians, 1988; DeHovitz, 1990; Northfelt et al., 1988). These physicians may agree that there is an obligation to treat those with HIV, but the evidence in most communities suggests that this perceived obligation may not extend to retaining primary care responsibility for them. It is not known whether private primary care physicians cease to see their HIV patients because the patients have no insurance, because the physicians are afraid of the risk of contagion or of losing their other patients, or because they are uncertain about their clinical skills. However, the comment made repeatedly in each of the 15 communities studied in the RWJF evaluation is that only a handful of private physicians are seeing the vast majority of persons with HIV disease. The public sector is similarly constrained.

A related issue is the availability of dental care for persons with HIV disease in many communities across the country. The topic of access to dental care has been hotly debated for several years. Thus, it is difficult to separate access barriers due to fear of spreading the disease from the low levels of access to dental care in this population (Capilouto et al., 1991; Neidle, 1989; Vercusio et al., 1989).

Despite these concerns for the future, the gap in availability of medical and nursing care was not given the highest priority among health and social service providers in RWJF-funded communities. More important, they felt, was the absence of housing and inadequate funding for home nursing, attendant services, and subacute long-term care facilities. Future demand for health services, and its potential for compromising access by outstripping the existing supply of physicians and clinic slots, will have to be carefully monitored and probably will vary considerably from community to community and by risk group.

Personal Barriers

This category of barriers includes those factors traditionally associated with differential access, regardless of disease or age—for example, education, ethnicity, or income. Historically, these factors have been shown to influence the behavior of providers in treating patients and the ability of patients to adhere to a prescribed treatment regimen. These personal characteristics tend to be correlated with socioeconomic status, making it difficult to disentangle the effects of personal characteristics from the effects of living in a particular neighborhood, the lack of insurance coverage, and reliance on public medical resources for medical care.

One clear indicator of access to care is whether infected individuals who should be receiving a given therapy are actually receiving it. Holmberg and colleagues (1990) found that as many as half of all AIDS patients were not receiving aerosolized pentamidine when it was the therapy of choice. In the RWJF AHSP evaluation sample, among those eligible to receive aerosolized pentamidine, men were four times as likely as women to have received it. This finding held true after controlling for disease duration, drug use, and insurance status, all of which were also significantly related to treatment (Piette et al., in press). Hidalgo and colleagues (1990) also found a surprisingly small number in the Maryland Medical or Pharmacy Assistance program on pentamidine. Findings on who received the drug were similar to those in the RWJF study: those more likely to have received the drug were gay, white men.

Another drug known to be of benefit to persons with HIV disease is

AZT (zidovudine). Since 1987, when it was shown to be effective in prolonging survival in patients with advanced disease, the federal and state governments have invested heavily in making this drug available to the infected population (Buchanan, 1988). But there is evidence that certain subgroups of the AIDS population are less likely than others to receive this treatment. Moore and colleagues (1991) studied the files of 714 adults in Maryland diagnosed with AIDS and found that women, minorities, and intravenous drug users were less likely to have received AZT than were gay, white men, even after controlling for ability to pay and access to a regular source of care at a clinic. Study data showed that 63 percent of white patients had received AZT, compared with only 43 percent of nonwhite patients. A similar pattern was observed for receipt of AZT among clinically eligible clients of the RWJF evaluation survey (Stein et al., 1991). After controlling for disease stage and past history of *Pneumocystis carinii* pneumonia, intravenous drug users, women, and minorities were significantly less likely to have received AZT than whites, males, and those with insurance. These effects remained as strong when the analyses were restricted to patients who receive their medical care from public hospital clinics.

Other utilization-based indicators of access differentials related to personal background have not been examined carefully for persons with HIV disease. The RWJF evaluation survey found that among persons served by the public hospital clinic, whites, those with more education, and non-drug users reported more frequent clinic visits in the past three months than the average patient, even after controlling for disease advance, symptom severity, functional status, and living arrangements (Mor et al., 1992). The opposite set of relationships was observed when the dependent variable was the likelihood of using an emergency room; use was more likely among minorities, women, and drug users.

Whether these differences signify reduced access to care must be carefully considered, because a greater number of visits does not necessarily translate into higher quality of care. Indeed, observed utilization differences do not imply provider bias; intravenous drug users may not have been socialized to, or have adopted, the norms of being compliant patients. Nevertheless, most public hospital clinics in the RWJF program reported high rates of missed appointments for clinic patients. If missed appointments were found disproportionately among minority and drug-using patients, it could explain their lower rate of use.

In conceptualizing utilization per se as an indicator of access, the value implications of "more is better" must be considered. It is not helpful to blame patients for noncompliance if they do not understand its importance. Yet even if public hospital systems could assume responsibility for ensuring patients' compliance, this orientation might engender unnecessary dependence. Some condition-specific approach that would leave less room for debate about values is probably necessary to determine whether more or less physician utilization is necessarily good or bad. At the same time, it must be recognized that not even this more restricted approach will reveal whether the observed differences in utilization arise from provider biases or from patients' insistence or noncompliance.

Attitudinal Barriers

The attitudes of providers can influence patient access to the personal health care system. This statement applies to primary care medicine, specialty medical or surgical care, dental care, hospital care, nursing home, and home health aide care. Because all of these health care providers are part of society in general, no discussion of access problems attributable to the attitudes of health care workers would be complete without considering broader societal messages and influences.

Societal reactions to the emergence of an infectious chronic disease that is fatal have varied considerably over the past decade, ranging from serious proposals for quarantining persons with HIV infection to massive voluntary efforts, both financial and otherwise, directed at providing support to those suffering from the disease (Blendon and Donelan, 1988; Brandt, 1988; Musto, 1986). These attitudes are reflected in the health care professions and influence patient access to the personal health care system. In addition, attitudes of non-HIV patients may play a role: the views of such patients about being treated by a health care provider who treats persons with HIV may affect provider attitudes and behavior. A recent random sample survey of the U.S. population found that 25 percent of the public would stop seeing their doctor if they knew that their physician was also treating an HIV-infected person (Gerbert et al., 1989). Perhaps attitudinal barriers, as much as economic, structural, and personal barriers, can be assumed to influence the behavior of health care professionals, and to therefore play a subtle role in reducing access.

A substantial amount of research has been devoted to examining the attitudes of health care professionals and their willingness to treat persons with HIV infection. These topics were addressed in a disproportionately large number of social science abstracts at the fifth and sixth international AIDS conferences. A wide array of attitude surveys have been devised to measure fears, attitudes, and thoughts about working with persons who have HIV disease (Bernstein et al., 1990; Damrosch et al., 1990; Emanuel, 1988; Gordin et al., 1987; Kelly et al, 1987; MacDowell, 1989; McGrory et al., 1990; Merrill et al., 1989; Richardson et al., 1987; Shultz et al., 1988). The major categories of providers who have served as subjects for this research are physicians, residents, and medical students—as distinct from nurses and nursing students. Finally, a limited degree of research has focused on the policies and practices of institutions such as nursing homes and home health agencies.

Merrill and colleagues (1989) classified the concerns of physicians and students about working with persons with AIDS into three groups: fear of contagion, homophobia, and discomfort with dying patients. McGrory and coworkers (1990) surveyed medical students at Columbia University and found low levels of homophobia but high rates of prejudice against treating intravenous drug users. Kelly and others (1987) surveyed physicians in three major cities asking about prejudice and willingness to interact socially with similar patients but under two disease scenarios: AIDS versus leukemia. In contrast to their view of leukemia patients, respondents saw AIDS patients as responsible for their illness and dangerous to others; they also indicated that they would experience greater discomfort in socializing with AIDS patients than with leukemia patients.

Negative attitudes about working with HIV-infected individuals also reflect broader social biases. The role of religious and moral beliefs as influences on the attitudes of health care providers' toward people with HIV has also been investigated. Francis (1989) assessed religiously based moral beliefs about AIDS and compared black and white clergy, medical students, and physicians as well as a sample of the public in the South. The disquieting results suggested that a majority of rural whites outside the health professions believe that HIV is a divine retribution and that 1 in 10 responding physicians feel this way.

Fear of contagion is another critical factor that may influence provider behavior. The survey by Kelly and coworkers (1987) suggested that fear of contagion was a central theme underlying physicians' negative attitudes toward AIDS patients. Educational programs targeting health professionals appear to be effective, both in increasing knowledge of the practices necessary to avoid infection and in changing behavior (Muskin and Stevens, 1990). However, they appear to have a differential impact on medical and dental students, with medical students more likely than dental students to manifest positive changes in attitude (Bernstein et al., 1990). Yet even after exposure to a training program, one-third of medical students and two-thirds of dental students said that they did not want to select a specialty that would bring them into contact with a high percentage of AIDS patients during their training. The authors suggest that these anxieties may influence the career choices of such students. Indeed, the study by Merrill and colleagues (1989) found that fear was the biggest factor in students' not wanting to work with HIV-infected patients. Several studies have noted that practicing physicians, house staff, students, and nursing staff all appear to have considerable skepticism about experts' assurances that they have a low probability of becoming infected (Francis, 1989; Wallack, 1989). Wallack found that this lack of trust was greatest among minority staff.

Several surveys have investigated the attitudes of nurses toward caring for HIV-infected patients. These studies generally reveal that the attitudes of nurses and nursing students are far more favorable toward AIDS patients than those of the general public. Variations in nurses' and nursing students' attitudes and fears about working with HIV-infected patients appear to be related to their knowledge of HIV transmission and their prior contact with patients (Gordin et al., 1987). Damrosch and colleagues (1990) surveyed critical care nurses in a teaching hospital and a denominational community hospital and found that teaching hospital nurses had more favorable attitudes than other nurses. Nonetheless, these authors reported that, given a choice, many of these nurses (45 percent in the teaching and 65 percent in the community hospital) would refuse to care for persons with AIDS.

Interestingly, although 26 percent of staff at a New York City teaching hospital felt that they would become infected with HIV and develop AIDS as a result of occupational exposure, 97 percent were nevertheless committed to continuing to care for these patients. This apparently contradictory finding means that interpreting attitudinal information without also investigating how health care professionals actually behave could result in incorrect, excessively pessimistic interpretations. Judgments of the impact of attitudes on access to health care for HIV-infected individuals must rely on more than surveys of knowledge and attitudes. The literature suggests that attitudes and a sense of comfort in caring for AIDS patients improve with educational exposure and time. Yet health care workers seem to remain anxious about infection and might elect not to run the risk of exposure, were they not committed to their jobs and professions. The behavior of interest, however, is whether health care workers refuse to treat HIV-infected patients if asked to do so. To date, there have been only limited instances of this phenomenon in the health care field, particularly once institutional and professional leaders set the pace.

Compared with the large number of attitudinal studies, relatively little research addresses institutional policies regarding the treatment of AIDS patients. The major medical societies have explicit policy statements on the responsibility of physicians to treat patients with HIV disease (AMA Council on Ethical and Judicial Affairs, 1988; Emanuel, 1988). There is apparently no consensus among the membership, however, and some studies suggest that between one-quarter and one-half of all physicians feel they have the right to refuse to treat some patients (Merrill et al., 1989; Rizzo et al., 1990).

Early in the epidemic, most hospitals established policies that prohibited staff from refusing to care for patients with HIV disease (McCarthy, 1988). In major metropolitan areas, most hospitals have served HIV-infected patients. With the increasing dehospitalization of HIV care, the establishment of specialty units for the tertiary care of complex and advanced cases of HIV disease, such as already occurs for cancer, may be seriously entertained. Evidence that patient outcomes are improved and that resources are more effectively used when care is provided by experienced hospitals suggests that such proposals may have merit (Bennett et al., 1990). In New York, there have been calls to establish specialty medical facilities, in both subacute and acute care settings, for the exclusive treatment of patients with HIV disease (Mayor's Task Force on AIDS, 1989; Weinberg, 1990). Rothman and Tynan (1990) reviewed many of the advantages of separate facilities as well as the historical evidence for not using segregation as a way of improving quality, and they strongly advocate an integrated approach to mainstreaming patients with HIV disease. An argument for this position is that if specialty facilities become the strategy to ensure rational allocation of responsibility for care, it would be impossible to differentiate the desirable practice of specialization from the undesirable practice of discriminating against patients with HIV disease by deflecting them to other facilities.

In a recent study by Fleishman and Masterson-Allen (1991) of home health agencies in 11 cities with high AIDS prevalence, executives of agencies that have served HIV patients were asked to respond to an open-ended telephone interview regarding their experiences. Staff stress was a problem associated with treating persons with AIDS, but the stresses tended to relate to the complexity of patients' nursing needs and the severity of their illness rather than to fear of contagion or to prejudices. In almost all cases, agencies developed specific policies about caring for patients with HIV disease and implemented management policies that prohibited staff from refusing to work with these patients.

In contrast, nursing homes have not encouraged the acceptance of HIV-infected patients. A survey of nursing homes in Ohio found that none had actually treated an HIV-infected patient and that only 25 percent would even consider admitting such a patient (MacDowell, 1989). Most felt that specialized facilities, such as those being fostered in New York, were the most appropriate setting for these patients. Administrators expressed concerns about possibly losing both staff and current residents if AIDS patients were admitted. These results were consistent with the reaction of the nursing home industry in general.

VIABILITY OF DEVELOPING ACCESS INDICATORS FROM EXISTING DATA SETS

Ideally, social indicators should be derived easily from routinely gathered statistics. Age- and sex-adjusted mortality ratios of blacks and whites are an example of such indicators, as are hospital discharge rates per 100,000 persons in certain age-sex groups for given diagnostic conditions. Indicators of access to the personal health care system are not as easily available, however, particularly for the relatively rare condition of HIV disease.

This section proposes indicators of barriers to health care access for persons with HIV disease consistent with the three goals outlined by the IOM committee: (1) avoiding premature mortality from diseases amenable to early case-finding; (2) avoiding premature mortality from life-threatening conditions for which effective medical management exists; and (3) providing services that reduce morbidity or improve functioning. Indicators might be derived from existing, ongoing data systems that are already in place, special-purpose merges of normally unlinked data systems, and surveys of the population that should contain samples of persons with HIV disease.

Decreased Mortality Using Case-Finding

Before the advent of effective antiviral treatments to increase survival, any discussion of HIV testing was largely influenced by concerns about confidentiality. It may therefore seem strange, given the debate over the past decade about "anonymous" versus "voluntary" testing, to use HIV testing as an indicator of access to care. But antiviral therapy is now advocated early in the course of disease. In view of available life-prolonging therapeutics, those who are at risk and who are not tested are at a disadvantage. Early case-finding is as important for HIV disease as it is for breast and cervical cancer. Just as use of mammography is a "utilization"-based indicator of access to the personal health care system that is relevant for breast cancer, it is now reasonable to use the rate of HIV testing in the population as a utilization indicator of access.

Measures of the testing rate per 1,000 persons within age-sex-race profiles, using aggregated data from anonymous test sites, should provide an indication of the level of "access" to early identification for each population subgroup. In states such as Colorado, where HIV infection is a reportable condition, the rate of testing could be calculated after removing from the denominator the number of people in that subpopulation who are already infected.

The measurement task is not a simple one, however, because a myriad of conceptual and technical complications are associated with using such data as the basis for examining differential access. First, in many states, testing is available outside of state-operated anonymous test sites in settings that still protect anonymity. In addition, anecdotal evidence points to considerable out-of-state travel, particularly from states that have aggressive partner notification programs, to secure even greater anonymity in testing. Moreover, estimates of the at-risk population, whether gay men or intravenous drug users, are notoriously inaccurate; this means that the denominators for these rates would have to be calculated separately for various age, sex, and racial groups. It also implies a recognition that the numerators (the number of people tested in each group) might reflect many persons from outside the geographic population base of interest.

Screening programs for treatable conditions are considered effective if there is evidence that they are used by a large unbiased proportion of the population or if there is evidence of a reduction in the rate at which the disease is identified in a later, untreatable stage. As applied to HIV disease, there are several potential indicators of the success of an early identification program. One example relies on the existing CDC-maintained national AIDS "registry" of all cases reported by each state's department of health. In addition to data on risk group and presenting diseases, the registry includes data on mortality. One class of deaths includes those that occur within the same calendar quarter in which the case was reported. Early identification programs should reduce the prevalence of such cases in registries.

Another example of an outcome indicator of early identification programs is the proportion of first admissions for HIV-related conditions that occur in late stages. Turner and her colleagues (1989) have developed a staging system for AIDS, based on hospital diagnoses, that predicts in-hospital mortality. By using linked hospital discharge abstract record systems such as exist in New York, it is possible to identify an individual's first HIV-related hospitalization. By applying a disease staging system, the rate of presentation with advanced HIV disease at first hospitalization can be determined.

Several conceptual and methodological limitations and constraints must be considered in evaluating the validity of these outcome indicators. With respect to the AIDS registry, a host of concerns arise about reporting biases and the completeness of case ascertainment and mortality follow-up. Furthermore, case reporting for AIDS is based on an arbitrary set of clinical symptoms identified early in the epidemic. There has already been one change in the definition of AIDS that complicated use of the registry for epidemiological purposes. The designation of AIDS implies presumptive eligibility for total disability under the SSDI (Social Security Disability Insurance) program, meaning that an AIDS diagnosis represents an entitlement for financial and other benefits. Given the underrepresentation of opportunistic infections concentrated among women in the AIDS case definition criteria, there is now considerable pressure to change the definition again. Obviously, any such change will alter the validity of indicators based on the registry and will limit longitudinal comparisons.

Certain states (e.g., New York, California, Massachusetts, Maryland) have statewide, uniform hospital discharge abstract reporting systems that include information on the charges or costs incurred per discharge, in addition to information on length of stay, discharge diagnoses, and payer source. New York has assembled the Statewide Planning and Research Cooperative System (SPARCS), which links the discharges of individuals, thus facilitating historical analyses of changes in an individual's payment sources and diagnoses (Kaufman et al., 1990). This diagnostic data set can be used to determine whether a patient's first HIV-related hospitalization occurs during an early or late stage of the disease. This estimate can be aggregated to the county or catchment area level to characterize the effectiveness of early identification programs in given locales.

The validity of measures derived from systems like the SPARCS as indicators of late diagnosis can be undermined by rapidly changing patterns of care; for example, increasing emphasis on outpatient treatment, both at home and in clinics, may lead to the avoidance of hospitalization for some patients. Thus, relying only on hospital-based statistical indicators under this scenario will confuse newly diagnosed with end-stage, drug-using patients.

Reduced Mortality Using Medical Management

Among the indicators of appropriate utilization of services that are assumed to address the overall goal of mortality reduction is the receipt of therapeutics that are known to affect survival. Consensus has been reached on the soundness of the evidence showing the effectiveness of retroviral drugs and antimicrobial agents, both in response to illness and for prophylaxis. Utilization-based indicators of access should be based on the rate of use of these drugs in various subgroups of the population. These rates can be derived from special statewide merged data sets such as the HIV Information System in Maryland, which links health department AIDS reporting information with Medicaid and Blue Cross/Blue Shield claims (including pharmaceuticals) and with hospital discharge abstracts (Hidalgo, 1990).

Another approach, which was used in the evaluation of the RWJF multicity project, is to survey individuals about their receipt of these treatments. The Agency for Health Care Policy and Research (AHCPR) has funded the AIDS Cost and Services Utilization Survey (ACSUS), which is currently in the field. The survey asks respondents about their use of AIDS-related therapeutics and will be abstracting comparable data from physician and hospital records.

Reliance on specialized data bases and surveys requires knowing well in advance the information that needs to be collected. Changes in the types of drugs being used and in how they are reimbursed may undermine the accuracy and validity of these types of indicators unless a mechanism can be developed for continuous updating of treatment-related information. For example, a new drug may be introduced and rapidly disseminated among treating physicians while a survey is in the field; without a mechanism to capture such a change in treatment, the effects of the drug may be missed and the validity of the earlier target treatments (which are replaced by the new one) as access indicators will be undermined. Special merged data sets may be similarly compromised, particularly if a lag occurs between acceptance in the field of the new treatment's effectiveness and the treatment's acceptance by insurers, particularly public insurers, as a reimbursable claim.

The outcome of access to medical management, including antiviral treatment, should be to increase survival. In spite of the limitations of the national CDC registry, it is an appropriate vehicle by which to examine this issue. However, an adjustment must be made for the effect of late-stage diagnosis, since prior to diagnosis the disease could not have been managed. Thus, survival differentials among those who live at least three to six months postdiagnosis are a potential indicator of access.

Although these comparisons are broadly applicable, there is reason to believe that survival differentials are related not merely to differences in medical management but also to the health status of the host and the efficiency of the mode of transmission of the virus. Intravenous drug users, for instance, may have compromised their health before being exposed to HIV. In addition, transmission by contaminated needles, rather than sexually, may be much more efficient at spreading the virus within an organism. Consequently, the mere comparison of survival rates among risk groups, after adjusting for late-diagnosed cases, could overstate the effects of medical management. Use of a special-purpose merged data system, such as the one in Maryland, makes it possible to statistically control for differences in risk groups and to assess the effects of treatment across all risk groups through stratified analyses (Moore et al., 1991).

Reduced Morbidity and Improved Function

Providing of services that reduce morbidity and improve functioning is often considered synonymous with out-of-hospital care. Evidence from a number of studies of persons with AIDS suggests a strong preference for care at home and for maintaining control over medical decisionmaking (Teno et al., 1990, 1992). Thus, it is safe to say that this population values time spent at home and away from the hospital.

Examples of utilization indicators of access to services that can help reduce morbidity include the rate of hospital admissions through the emergency room, the proportion of people with AIDS who use home health agency services, and the number of additional days spent in the hospital due to administrative discharge delays. Data on home health use must be derived from periodic surveys of the population such as the ACSUS. Hospital admissions through the emergency room and the number of administrative, or "outlier," days can be obtained from the National Center for Health Statistics (NCHS), which maintains ongoing data on a large number of hospital discharge abstracts used to estimate population-level hospital use rates by discharge diagnosis.

Considerable care must be taken in interpreting the meaning of admission through the emergency room and extended hospital stays, since the medical care system is not necessarily the most efficient structure for redressing other societal inequities (e.g., limited social support and financial resources for intravenous drug users, lack of drug treatment program openings that could facilitate their discharge). Moreover, in many parts of the country, physicians instruct patients to enter the hospital through the emergency room, reflecting a hospital operating strategy. Because it is likely that hospitals in different areas use their emergency rooms in very different fashions, differences in rates of emergency room use by subgroups may reflect administrative styles and not merely access differences.

Outcome indicators of access associated with the goal of reducing morbidity can be conceived of as avoiding unnecessary hospitalization and receiving care at home. The first of these can be measured by using a population-based uniform hospital discharge abstract system matched with a statewide AIDS registry at the zip code, or census tract, level. The registry data provide the denominator of AIDS cases, and the hospital discharge abstracts provide the numerator of admissions for specific conditions, such as *Pneumocystis carinii* pneumonia (PCP). Rates of PCP-related hospitalization for minorities and nonminorities can be compared on the assumption that effective prophylactic treatment would minimize hospitalization.

A methodological limitation of the validity of this measure involves the transience of patients: many will not necessarily continue receiving care in a single hospital. Patients' addresses on discharge abstracts are often coded geographically by zip code or census tract; matching these codes with comparably coded registry information is problematic because either address may be incorrect, particularly among certain groups. Naturally, this bias would undermine the validity of any comparison.

Since 1987, when uniform coding of AIDS with the *International Classification of Diseases-9* framework began for hospital discharge and for vital and health statistics, death certificates have offered another source of data from which selected indicators can be derived. Among HIV disease-related deaths, the distribution of the location of death can be examined. As of 1989, the nationally standardized death certificate coding scheme has included a data element for deaths occurring at home as opposed to in the hospital, in a nursing home or at another site. Those AIDS patients who die at home could be compared on the basis of gender, age, race, and geographic area as an indicator of the availability and use of home health and out-of-hospital services.

Much health and social policymaking over the past several years has been devoted to buttressing community support services to reduce reliance on hospital care. Recently, McMillan and colleagues (1990) demonstrated that policies on hospices have affected the site of death of Medicare beneficiaries dying of cancer; the study used Medicare claims merged with death certificates. Some evidence suggests that AIDS patients also would prefer to die at home (Teno et al., 1992). Consequently, the proportion of deaths that occur at home can be a useful barometer of access to services that is particularly applicable when looking at age- and sex-adjusted rates within certain metropolitan areas known to have strong home support services.

CONCLUSION

Despite the promise of the various data systems that have been suggested as the basis for deriving access indicators, the rapidly changing circumstances of the epidemic, the variability in state programs offering subsidized or free care to the poor, and the regional variation in Medicaid coverage make it difficult to imagine a data system that would have complete disease, health utilization, and outcome data on a representative sample of persons with HIV. Consequently, even given a better understanding of the meaning of the suggested indicators, the result is likely to be a series of incomplete snapshots. Each will have its own limitations and biases of which users, particularly policymakers, must be aware. Yet despite these limitations, many of the merged data system files proposed above hold considerable promise and should be explored further. By "cross walking" findings from the more detailed surveys, such as ACSUS, with the population-based utilization estimates derived from merged data systems, a more informed opinion could be obtained about the validity of the resulting access indicators. Ideally, when indicators such as those suggested here are assembled into a montage, they will form a more coherent, more consistent picture.

REFERENCES

AMA (American Medical Association) Council on Ethical and Judicial Affairs. 1988. Ethical issues involved in the growing AIDS crisis. *Journal of the American Medical Association* 259:1360-1361.

American College of Physicians, Health and Public Policy Committee, and the Infectious Diseases Society of America. 1988. The acquired immunodeficiency syndrome (AIDS) and infection with the human immunodeficiency virus (HIV). *Annals of Internal Medicine* 258:2714-2717.

Andrulis, D. P. 1989. *Crisis at the Frontline.* New York, NY: The Twentieth Century Fund, p. 50.

Andrulis, D. P., Beers, V. S., Bentley, J. D., et al. 1987a. The provision and financing of medical care for AIDS patients in U.S. public and private teaching hospitals. *Journal of the American Medical Association* 258:1343-1346.

Andrulis, D. P., Beers, V. S., Bentley, J. D., and Gage, L. S. 1987b. State Medicaid policies and hospital care for AIDS patients. *Health Affairs* (Winter)6:110-118.

Andrulis, D. P., Weslowski, V. B., and Gage, L. S. 1989. The 1987 U.S. Hospital AIDS survey. *Journal of the American Medical Association* 262:784-794.

Arno, P. S., Shenson, D., Siegel, N. F., Franks, P., and Lee, P. R. 1990. Economic and policy implications of early intervention in HIV disease. *Journal of the American Medical Association* 262:1493-1499.

Baily, M. A., Bilheimer, L., Wooldridge, J., Langwell, K., and Greenberg, W. 1990. Economic consequences for Medicaid of human immunodeficiency virus infection. *Health Care Financing Review* 12:97-108.

Benjamin, A. E. 1988. Long term care and AIDS: Perspectives from experience with the elderly. *Milbank Quarterly* 66:415-443.

Bennett, C. L., Gertler, P., Guze, P. A., Garfinkle, J. B., Kanouse, D. E., and Greenfield, S. 1990. The relation between resource use and in-hospital mortality for patients with acquired immunodeficiency syndrome related *Pneumocystis carinii* pneumonia. *Archives of Internal Medicine* 150:1447-1452.

Bernstein, C. A., Tabkin, J. G., and Wolland, H. J. 1990. Medical and dental students' attitudes about AIDS issues. *Academic Medicine* 65:458-460.

Blendon, R. J. and Donelan, K. 1988. Discrimination against people with AIDS: The public's perspective. *New England Journal of Medicine* 319:1022-1026.

Brandt, A. M. 1988. AIDS in historical perspective: Four lessons from the history of sexually transmitted diseases. *American Journal of Public Health* 78:367-371.

Buchanan, R. J. 1988. State Medicaid coverage of AZT and AIDS-related policies. *American Journal of Public Health* 78:432-436.

Capilouto, E. I., Piette, J., White, B. A., and Fleishman, J. 1991. Perceived need for dental care among persons living with acquired immunodeficiency syndrome. *Medical Care* 29:745-754.

CDC (Centers for Disease Control). 1990. HIV prevalence estimates and AIDS case projections for the United States: Report based upon a workshop. *Morbidity and Mortality Weekly Report* 39(RR-16):1-31.

CDC (Centers for Disease Control). 1991. Mortality attributable to HIV infection/AIDS—United States, 1981-1990. *Morbidity and Mortality Weekly Report* 40:41-44.

Cohen, P. T., Sande, M. A., and Volberding, P. 1990. *The AIDS Knowledge Base.* Waltham, Mass.: Medical Publishing Group.

Damrosch, S., Abbey, S., Warner, A., and Guy, S. 1990. Critical care nurses' attitudes toward, concerns about, and knowledge of the acquired immunodeficiency syndrome. *Heart-Lung* 19:395-400.

DeHovitz, J. A. 1990. The increasing role of primary care in the management of HIV-infected patients. *New York State Journal of Medicine* 90:119-120.

Eby, C. 1989. The share of AIDS medical care costs paid by private insurance in the United States. P. 1047 in Abstracts from the Fifth International Conference on AIDS, Montreal, Quebec, June 4–9. Abstract T.H.P. 24. Ottawa: International Development Research Centre.

Emanuel, E. 1988. Do physicians have an obligation to treat patients with AIDS? *New England Journal of Medicine* 315:1686-1690.

Faden, R. R. and Kass, N. E. 1988. Health insurance and MDs: The status of state regulatory activity. *American Journal of Public Health Statistics* 78:437-438.

Fischl, M. A., Richman, D. D., Grieco, M. H., et al. 1987. The efficacy of azidothymidine (AZT) in the treatment of patients with AIDS and AIDS-related complex: A double-blind, placebo-controlled trial. *New England Journal of Medicine* 317:185-191.

Fleishman, J. 1990. Research issues in service integration and coordination. Pp. 167-187 in *Community-Based Care for Persons with AIDS: Developing a Research Agenda,* AHCPR

Conference Proceedings. DHHS Pub. No. (PHS)90-3456. Rockville, Md.: U.S. Government Printing Office.

Fleishman, J. A., Cwi, J., and Mor, V. 1989. Sampling and accessing people with AIDS: A study of program clients in nine locations. Pp. 181-186 in Proceedings of the Fifth Conference on Health Survey Research Methods, Floyd J. Fowler (ed.). DHHS Pub. No. (PHS)89-3447. Washington, D.C.: U.S. Government Printing Office.

Fleishman, J. A., and Masterson-Allen, S. 1991. Delivery of home care to people with AIDS. Final report prepared for the Agency for Health Care Policy and Research.

Fleishman, J. A., Mor, V., and Piette, J. 1991. AIDS case management: The client's perspective. *Health Services Research* 26(Oct.):447-470.

Fleishman, J. A., Piette, J., and Mor, V. 1990. Organizational response to AIDS. *Evaluation and Program Planning* 13:31-38.

Francis, R. A. 1989. Moral beliefs of physicians, medical students, clergy, and lay public concerning AIDS. *Journal of the National Medical Association* 81:1141-1147.

Gerbert, B., Maquire, B. T., Hulley, S. B., and Coates, T. J. 1989. Physicians and acquired immunodeficiency syndrome: What patients think about human immunodeficiency virus in medical practice. *Journal of the American Medical Association* 262:1969-1972.

Ginzberg, J. 1990. *Health Services Research: Key to Health Policy*. Cambridge, Mass.: Harvard University Press.

Gordin, F., et al. 1987. Knowledge of AIDS among hospital workers: Behavioral correlates and consequences. *Journal of Acquired Immune Deficiency Syndromes* 1:183-188.

Green, J. and Arno, P. S. 1990. The Medicaidization of AIDS: Trends in the financing of HIV-related medical care. *Journal of the American Medical Association* 264:1261-1266.

Harris, J. E. 1990. Improved short term survival of AIDS patients initially diagnosed with *Pneumocystic carinii* pneumonia. *Journal of the American Medical Association* 263:397-401.

Hayward, R. A., Bernard, A. M., Freeman, H. E., and Corey, C. R. 1991. Regular source of ambulatory care and access to health services. *American Journal of Public Health* 81:434-438.

Hidalgo, J., Sugland, B., Bareta, J. C., Allen, N., Moore, R. and Chaisson, R. E. 1990. Access, Equity, and Survival: Use of Zidovudine (ZVD) and Pentamidine by Persons with AIDS. Paper presented at the Sixth International Conference on AIDS, San Francisco, California, June 23.

Hidalgo, J. 1990. Development and application of statewide acquired immunodeficiency syndrome (AIDS) information systems in health services planning and evaluation. *Evaluation and Program Planning* 13:39-46.

Holahan, J. 1984. Paying for physician services in state Medicaid programs. *Health Care Financing Review* 5:99-110.

Holmberg, S. D., Harrison, J. S., Buckbinder, et al. 1990. Therapeutic and Prophylactic Drug Use by Homosexual and Bisexual Men in Three U.S. Cities. Paper presented at the Sixth Conference on AIDS, San Francisco, California, June 23.

IOM (Institute of Medicine). 1986. *Confronting AIDS*. Washington, D.C.: National Academy Press.

Kaplowitz, L. G., Turshen, J., Myers, P. S., Staloch, L. A., Berry, A. J., and Settle, J. T. 1988. Medical care costs of patients with acquired immunodeficiency syndrome in Richmond, VA: A quantitative analysis. *Archives of Internal Medicine* 148:1793-1797.

Kass, N. 1989. Access to insurance and perceived discrimination by homosexual men. P. 1047 in Abstracts from the Fifth International Conference on AIDS, Montreal, Quebec, June 4–9. Abstract T.H.P. 20. Ottawa: International Development Research Centre.

Kaufman, G. I., Grabau, J. C., Schmidt, E. M., and Han, Y. 1990. HIV infected hospital patients in New York city state. The development of longitudinal information from a hospital discharge data system. *New York State Journal of Medicine* 90:238-242.

Kelly, J. A., St. Lawrence, J. S., Smith, S., Hood, H. V., and Cook, D. J. 1987. Medical students' attitudes toward AIDS and homosexual patients. *Journal of Medical Education* 62:549-556.

Lemp, G. F., Payne, S. F., Neal, D. Temelso, T., and Rutherford, G. W. 1990. Survival trends for patients with AIDS. *Journal of the American Medical Association* 263:402-406.

Lipson, B. 1988. A crisis in insurance. *New England Journal of Public Policy* 285-305, Winter/Spring.

MacDowell, N. M. 1989. Willingness to provide care to AIDS patients in Ohio nursing homes. *Journal of Community Health* 14:205-213.

Marder, R. E. and Linsk, N. L. 1990. Assessment of discharge planning referral to nursing homes for people with AIDS and HIV. P. 287 in Abstracts from the Fifth International Conference on AIDS, Montreal, Quebec, June 4–9. Vol. 3, Abstract No. S.D. 791. Ottawa: International Development Research Centre.

Martin, C., Tortolero, S., Hines, A., Jardin, L., and Johnson, C. 1989. How do persons with symptomatic HIV disease finance their care in Texas? P. 1047 in Abstracts from the Fifth International Conference on AIDS, Montreal, Quebec, June 4–9. Abstract No. T.H.P. 22. Ottawa: International Development Research Centre.

Mayor's Task Force on AIDS. 1989. Assuring care for New York City's AIDS population. New York, N.Y.: Mayor's Task Force on AIDS, March.

McCarthy, C. 1988. The role of the American Hospital Association in combating AIDS. *Public Health Reports* 103:273-277.

McGrory, B. J., McDowell, D. M., and Muskin, P. R. 1990. Medical students' attitudes toward AIDS, homosexual and intravenous drug-abusing patients: A re-evaluation in New York City. *Psychosomatics* 31:426-433.

McMillan, A., Mentnech, R. M., Lubitz, J., McBean, A. M. and Russell, D. 1990. Trends and patterns in place of death for Medicare enrollees. *Health Care Financing Review* 12:1-7.

Mechanic, D. and Aiken, L. H. 1989. Lessons from the past: Responding to the AIDS crisis. *Health Affairs* 8(Fal):16-32.

Merrill, J. M., Laux, L., and Thornby, J. I. 1989. AIDS and student attitudes. *Southern Medical Journal* 82:426-432.

Moore, R. D., Hidalgo, J., Sugland, B. W., and Chaisson, R. E. 1991. Zidovudine and the natural history of the acquired immunodeficiency syndrome. *New England Journal of Medicine* 324:1412-1416.

Mor, V., Piette, J., and Fleishman, J. A. 1989. Community-based case management for persons with AIDS. *Health Affairs* 8(Winter):139-153.

Mor, V., Fleishman, J. A., Dresser, M., and Piette, J. 1992. Variation in health service use among HIV-infected patients. *Medical Care* 30:17-29.

Muskin, P. R. and Stevens, L. A. 1990. An AIDS educational program for third year medical students. *General Hospital Psychiatry* 12:390-395.

Musto, D. F. 1986. Quarantine and the problem of AIDS. *Milbank Memorial Fund Quarterly* 64(suppl. 1):97-117.

Myers, L. P., and Vladeck, B. C. 1990. New York City's Hospital Occupancy Crisis: Caring for a Changing Population. A report from the Bigel Institute for Health Policy, United Hospital Fund of New York, 1988, and the New York State Governor's Statewide Anti-Drug Abuse Council. Anti-Drug Abuse Strategy Report.

Neidle, E. A. 1989. AIDS-related changes in dental practice. *Journal of Dental Education* 9:525-528.

Northfelt, D. W., Hayward, R. A., Shapiro, M. F. 1988. The acquired immune deficiency syndrome is a primary care disease. *Annals of Internal Medicine* 109:773-775.

Parmet, W. E. 1987. AIDS and the limits of discrimination law. *Law, Medicine, and Health Care* 15:61-72.

Perloff, J. D., Kletke, P. R., and Neckeman, K. M. 1987. Physicians' decisions to limit Medicaid participation: Determinants and policy implications. *Journal of Health Politics, Policy and Law* 12:221-235.

Pickett, N. A., Drewry, S. J., and Comer, E. L. 1990. AIDS: MetLife's experience. *Statistical Bulletin—Metropolitan Life Insurance Company* 71:2-9.

Piette, J., Fleishman, J. A., Dill, A., and Mor, V. 1990. A comparison of hospital and community case management programs for persons with AIDS. *Medical Care* 28:746-755.

Piette, J., Stein, M., Mor, V., Fleishman, J. A., Mayer, K., Wachtel, T., and Carpenter, C. In press. Patterns of secondary prophylaxis with aerosol pentamidine among persons with AIDS (letter). *Journal of Acquired Immune Deficiency Syndrome.*

Richardson, J. L., Lochner, T., McGuigan, K., and Levine, A. M. 1987. Physicians' attitudes and experience regarding the care of patients with acquired immunodeficiency syndrome (AIDS) and related disorders (ARC). *Medical Care* 25:675-685.

Rizzo, J. A., Marder, W. D., and Willke, R. J. 1990. Physician contact with and attitudes toward HIV-seropositive patients: Results from a national survey. *Medical Care* 28:251-260.

Rothman, D. J. and Tynan, E. A. 1990. Advantages and disadvantages of special hospitals for patients with HIV infection. *New England Journal of Medicine* 323:764-768.

Rowe, M. J. and Ryan, C. C. 1988. Comparing state-only expenditures for AIDS. *American Journal of Public Health* 78:424-429.

Seage, G. R., Landers, S., Lamb, G. A., and Epstein, A. M. 1990. Effect of changing patterns of care and duration of survival on the cost of treating the acquired immunodeficiency syndrome (AIDS). *American Journal of Public Health* 80:835-839.

Shultz, J. M., MacDonald, K. L., Heckert, K. A., and Osterholm, M. T. 1988. The Minnesota AIDS Physician Survey. *Minnesota Medicine* 71:277-283.

Stein, M. D., Piette, J., Mor, V., Wachtel, T. J., Fleishman, J. A., Mayer, K. H., and Carpenter, C. 1991. Differences in access to zidovudine (AZT) among symptomatic HIV-infected persons. *Journal of General Internal Medicine* 6:35-40.

Swan, J. H., Benjamin, E. A., and Lee, P. R. 1990. Resource use for AIDS care in nursing homes. P. 286 in Abstracts from the Fifth International Conference on AIDS, Vol. 3. Abstract F.D. 816.

Teno, J., Fleishman, J. A., Brock, D. W., and Mor, V. 1990. The use of formal prior directives among patients with HIV-related diseases. *Journal of General Internal Medicine* 5:490-494.

Teno, J. Fleishman, J. A., and Mor, V. 1992. AIDS patients' preferences for community-based care. Unpublished paper.

Turner, B. J., Kelly, J. V., and Ball, J. K. 1989. A severity classification system for AIDS hospitals. *Medical Care* 27:423-437.

Vercusio, A. C., Neidle, E. A., Nash, K. D., Silverman, S. Horowitz, A. M., and Wagner, K. S. 1989. The dentist and infectious diseases: A national survey of attitudes and behavior. *Journal of the American Dental Association* 118:553-562.

Volberding, P. A., Lagakos, S. W., and Koch, M. A. et al. 1990. Zidovudine in asymptomatic human immunodeficiency virus infection: A controlled trial in persons with fewer than 500 CD4-positive cells per cubic millimeter. *New England Journal of Medicine* 332:941-949.

Wallack, J. J. 1989. AIDS anxiety among health care professionals. *Hospital and Community Psychiatry* 40:507-510.

Weinberg, L. 1990. Bill would require states to raise Medicaid AIDS rates. *Modern Healthcare*, p. 17.

White, C. M. and Berger, M. C. 1991. Response of hospitals, skilled nursing facilities and home health agencies in Oregon to AIDS: Reports of nursing executives. *American Journal of Public Health* 81:495-496.

Yelin, E. H., Greenblatt, R. M., Hollander, H., and McMaster, J. R. 1991. The impact of HIV-related illness on employment. *American Journal of Public Health* 81:79-84.

Zucconi, S., Kingsley, L., Lave, J., and Ishii, E. 1989. Impact of insurance coverage on health care utilization for HIV infected persons: Results of a survey. P. 289 in Abstracts from the Fifth International Conference on AIDS, Vol. 3, Abstract S.D. 797.

B

Developing Indicators of Access to Care: Waiting Lists for Drug Abuse Treatment

Don C. Des Jarlais[1] and Samuel R. Friedman[2]

The epidemic of acquired immune deficiency syndrome (AIDS) and the most recent version of the "war on drugs" have drawn increased attention to the issue of "waiting lists": lists of persons who have applied for drug abuse treatment but for whom a treatment position is not presently available. These waiting lists are generally seen as a measure of unmet demand for drug abuse treatment. For instance, the expansion of drug abuse treatment to the point where waiting lists need not occur was one of the primary recommendations of the Presidential Commission on the Human Immunodeficiency Virus Epidemic (hereafter the Presidential Commission; 1988). The National Commission on AIDS[3] has also advocated sufficient expansion of drug abuse treatment programming to prevent waiting lists (see the Commission's press release of September 26, 1989).

---

[1]Don C. Des Jarlais is Director of the Medical Dependency Unit at the Beth Israel Medical Center.

[2]Samuel R. Friedman is Senior Principal Investigator at National Development and Research Institutes, Inc.

[3]The National Commission on AIDS was established by an act of Congress in 1989, after the final report and termination of the Presidential Commission on the Human Immunodeficiency Virus Epidemic. The National Commission differs from the Presidential Commission in that members were appointed by Congress as well as the President, and the designated task of the National Commission is to provide policy recommendations to both Congress and the executive branch. Other than these two differences, the present National Commission is the successor to the Presidential Commission as the national advisory body responsible for developing policy recommendations regarding AIDS.

There is no consensus, however, on the issue of waiting lists. As discussed later in this paper, some experts in the drug abuse field contend that current waiting lists do not represent unmet demand for drug abuse treatment but rather poor referral mechanisms among currently operating drug abuse treatment programs. Other experts contend that current waiting lists greatly underestimate the unmet demand for treatment. Still others concede that waiting lists exist but nonetheless argue that treatment programs should not be expanded to the point where waiting lists would not occur.

This paper examines the empirical literature and expert opinions on waiting lists for drug abuse treatment and critiques the concept of waiting lists as a measure of unmet demand for treatment. Data from the early 1970s, when waiting lists for drug abuse treatment were also used as a measure of unmet treatment demand (U.S. House of Representatives, 1972), are included to provide some historical perspective. The limited data on the relationship between the waiting experience and subsequent client experience in drug abuse treatment are also reviewed. Finally, some unpublished data on the behavior of persons while on waiting lists are presented.

METHODS

The development of techniques such as meta-analysis has greatly increased the analytic power of reviews of the scientific literature. Unfortunately, such techniques are not appropriate for examining the literature on waiting lists for drug abuse treatment. First, the number of studies addressing this issue is quite small. As one research group interested in the topic noted, "In spite of the increasing reports of the need to employ waiting lists, and their significance for the user and the treatment program, there is a virtual absence of research in this area, with the exception of those studies using waiting list controls" (Brown et al., 1989). Fewer than 15 studies were found through computerized literature searches in the MEDLARS, DIALOG, and PsychINFO[4] data bases with "waiting list" as a keyword. Most of the studies appeared in at least two of these three data bases, suggesting considerable overlap among them; such duplication also implied that additional computer searching was not likely to lead to many other articles or books. Interestingly, neither of the two most recent studies of the number of persons on waiting lists throughout the country was in these computerized literature data bases.

Many of the studies in the data bases were not relevant to this paper. A number of them recruited research subjects from among persons already enrolled in drug abuse treatment and then randomly assigned them to imme-

---

[4]MEDLARS, DIALOG, and PsychINFO are registered trademarks.

diate entry into an additional treatment component or to a waiting list control group that received the additional treatment component after the experimental group (e.g., Henik and Domino, 1975; Ingram and Salzberg, 1990). This is a powerful research design for assessing additional components to standard drug abuse treatment, but because the waiting list controls are already receiving some form of standard treatment, the data from these studies are not relevant to the question of waiting lists for initial entry into treatment.

The computer searches did identify a number of waiting list control studies for alcoholism treatment, smoking cessation treatment, and various types of psychotherapy. After a brief review of a number of these studies, however, the decision was made not to discuss them here. Attempting to bridge the many differences in specific research methods, as well as the differences in substantive content, would have meant a loss of focus for the present work. Only one study, involving subjects with both alcohol and other drug problems, was included because of its potential relevance to the argument that waiting lists can perform a useful screening function.

A telephone survey of eight experts in drug abuse treatment was conducted to try to find additional studies that were not in the computerized literature data bases. Some additional sources of useful information surfaced, but waiting list information was usually tangential to the main thrust of these studies, so it is not surprising that they were not coded for "waiting list" in the data bases. Although both the Presidential Commission on the Human Immunodeficiency Virus Epidemic and the National Commission on AIDS held hearings on waiting lists for drug abuse treatment, and the testimony at these hearings provided a good range of expert opinions on the subject, these hearings also illustrate the relative lack of scientific data on the subject.

This paper draws, as well, on the past personal experience of one of its authors (D. C. Des Jarlais) as a research scientist for the Division of Substance Abuse Services of the state of New York. Because of the size of the state drug abuse treatment system and the concentration of programs in New York City, waiting lists and the demand for treatment have been administratively studied in New York for almost 20 years. New York attempts to both eliminate double-counting in its waiting list compilation and to distinguish between those persons on waiting lists who are not yet in any treatment program and those persons already in treatment but waiting to transfer to another program. (As discussed later in this paper, there are also persons who operate drug abuse treatment programs in New York who believe that the waiting lists are artificial.)

Finally, this paper contains some unpublished data on the behavior of persons listed as waiting to enter drug abuse treatment. These data were collected as part of a study of an "interim" methadone clinic funded by the

Centers for Disease Control (CDC; Yancovitz et al., 1991). They were the only data that the authors could locate that included longitudinal urinalysis results from persons on a waiting list for entry into drug abuse treatment.

Because of the difficulties that we encountered in finding scientific data on waiting lists for drug abuse treatment, this paper is closer to an essay than the series of meta-analyses that we would have liked to perform. The paper, therefore, expresses our personal opinions rather than conclusions based on a substantial literature relevant to the topic.

THE NUMBER OF PERSONS ON WAITING LISTS

The National Association of State Alcohol and Drug Abuse Directors (NASADAD) conducts occasional surveys of its members regarding waiting lists for drug abuse treatment. The 1989 survey covered 43 states and showed a total of 66,000 persons on waiting lists (Institute of Medicine, 1990). NASADAD's series of surveys is one of the few nationwide studies to date of waiting lists for drug abuse treatment. Yet although the NASADAD information is clearly useful, there are severe methodological limitations to these data. First, the definition of the term *waiting list* is not standardized across states (and probably is not standardized within many states). Some programs may include an applicant on a waiting list after a simple telephone contact, others after a face-to-face contact, and still others only after a preadmission determination of program eligibility has been made. There is probably even more variation regarding when programs remove applicants from a waiting list. Some programs remove applicants immediately if they do not respond to one attempted contact by letter or telephone; others do so only after repeated attempts at contact. Other programs remove applicants after a fixed period of time following the first attempt at contact, whereas others wait until one (or more) scheduled intake appointments have been missed. Some programs remove applicants from a waiting list at regular intervals; others do so sporadically. Moreover, the extent to which corrections for double-counting (when a single applicant is on waiting lists for more than one program) or for transfers (when an applicant on one program's waiting list is currently receiving treatment at another program) were made at the state level, before the data were submitted to NASADAD, is not known.

The U.S. Conference of Mayors (1987) conducted a survey of 42 cities in 1987 and found waiting lists for drug abuse treatment in three-quarters of those municipalities. The average duration of time on waiting lists ranged from 7 to 26 weeks. This survey cannot be used to estimate the total number of persons on waiting lists nationwide, but it does confirm the other studies indicating the widespread use of waiting lists throughout the country.

The National Institute on Drug Abuse (NIDA) recently completed a survey of waiting lists at the request of the Office of National Drug Control Policy (Anita Lewis Gadzuk, public health analyst, Office of Applied Studies, Substance Abuse and Mental Health Services Administration, personal communication, March 1991). Known as the Drug Services Research Survey (DSRS), this study differed from previous NASADAD studies in several ways. First, for-profit as well as publicly funded programs were included. Second, information on program capacity, program utilization, and program costs was also obtained. Third, the DSRS utilized a sampling technique rather than attempting to obtain information from all programs. Questionnaires were mailed to 1,183 programs, followed by telephone interviews to complete the questionnaire. Site visits to a subsample of 120 programs were then conducted, and 20 client records were examined at each site. The DSRS study, however, did not eliminate double-counting or waiting list transfers from its data collection.

Preliminary data from the DSRS study suggest that at the time that the study was conducted, there were 530,000 treatment slots in the United States and 107,000 persons on waiting lists. Sixty-three percent of persons who had entered treatment spent one month or less on a waiting list; 37 percent waited longer than one month. The average utilization rate for all programs was 90 percent. Great variation in utilization rates was seen, however, ranging from 56 percent for inpatient programs to 97 percent for methadone maintenance programs.

No certain explanations were found for the differences between the NASADAD and the DSRS results (e.g., 66,000 versus 107,000, respectively, as the total number of persons on waiting lists). The two surveys differed not only in the time at which they were conducted (i.e., 1989 for the NASADAD survey versus 1990 for the DSRS) but also in the sampling frame and the methodology of data collection employed. As discussed later, the large difference in the size of the waiting lists is probably not attributable solely to inclusion of the for-profit drug treatment programs in the DSRS study.

"THERE ARE NO REAL WAITING LISTS FOR TREATMENT"

Even though both the NASADAD and the DSRS studies showed large numbers of persons on waiting lists for drug abuse treatment in the United States, some experts argue that these waiting lists do not represent unmet demand for treatment per se. Prominent among these is Dr. Beny Primm, who previously headed the Addiction Research and Treatment Corporation (ARTC), a large methadone maintenance treatment program in New York City. He is currently head of the Office of Treatment Improvement, a component agency of the federal Alcohol, Drug Abuse, and Mental Health

Administration. The major premise of Dr. Primm's argument is that waiting lists represent the drug treatment system's inability to efficiently refer persons applying for treatment to programs that have unused capacity. When he was at the ARTC and the program did not have places for new applicants, he found that calling other programs in the city would almost always identify a program with an open treatment slot (B. Primm, personal communication, March 1991). This was during a time, the late 1980s, when the official waiting list of persons applying for treatment in New York City averaged more than 1,000 individuals.[5]

The argument that the present treatment waiting lists represent poor treatment referral systems (and not unmet demand) is clearly a minority position—but it does deserve consideration. It is possible to reconcile Primm's experience at the ARTC with the waiting lists reported by other programs in New York. There are approximately 35,000 long-term drug abuse treatment positions in New York City, with a turnover of probably 20,000 persons per year.[6] Thus, diligent referral work can often locate an open position in a treatment program. Sometimes this slot will be found at a program that has openings and no current waiting list. Often, the open position will be one that had been assigned to a person on a waiting list for a "full" program but the applicant had failed to show up for the intake procedures. (The question of waiting list applicants who fail to appear for intake will be discussed in some detail later.)

Street outreach programs in New York City also report that they receive many requests for assistance in securing a place in a treatment program and that diligent referral work can locate an opening for many of these individuals (Centers for Disease Control, 1990; Des Jarlais 1989; Friedman et al., in press; Jackson and Rotkiewicz, 1987). These outreach programs also report, however, that the unmet demand for treatment is real and that the ability to find an opening for an individual client is quite a different matter from the ability to place the large numbers of persons who evidently want to enter drug abuse treatment. Within a large, high-turnover drug treatment system such as that in New York City, it is quite possible that better referral work could place a substantial number of additional individuals in treatment programs; yet it is also true that the waiting lists still reflect a substantial unmet need for treatment.

---

[5]The Office of Treatment Improvement has the responsibility of awarding grants for the federal monies appropriated to reduce waiting lists. Consistent with Dr. Primm's experience in New York, the grant to New York has primarily been allocated to establish a central intake and referral service rather than simply expanding the number of treatment positions.

[6]If one included the short-term detoxification programs in New York, the turnover in positions would be increased by another 5,000 to 10,000. The average length of stay in these publicly funded inpatient detoxification programs is less than one week.

At another level of analysis, quite good evidence exists that waiting lists and unused treatment capacity currently coexist in the United States. There are a large number of for-profit treatment programs in the nation, and many of them clearly have unused capacity. The DSRS study found that the average utilization rate among for-profit programs was only 57 percent. Indeed, the utilization rates of these programs are so low that many of them are in danger of closing (Korcok, 1991). However, within current drug abuse treatment systems in the United States, it would not be possible to reduce waiting lists by simply referring applicants from publicly funded programs to for-profit programs. The for-profit programs typically require that their clients have either private health insurance or the ability to pay the substantial fees that these programs charge.[7] McAuliffe (1990) has described the results of the two-tier (publicly and privately funded) structure of programs as having "rationed treatment to lower-income addicts seeking care."

The two parallel systems—of publicly funded and for-profit drug abuse treatment programs—are in many ways similar to the general provision of health care in the United States, and a detailed analysis of what would have to happen in order for persons on waiting lists for publicly funded programs to be accommodated within for-profit programs is beyond the scope of this paper. We merely note that integration of the programs would require a major philosophical change in the way drug abuse treatment is funded in this country. It would also require an open examination of the social class and ethnic/racial antagonisms that the present two-tier structure conceals.

WAITING LISTS UNDERESTIMATE UNMET DEMAND

The preceding section presented the arguments surrounding the notion that current waiting lists overestimate the unmet demand for drug abuse treatment. Yet there are also those who argue that current waiting lists substantially underestimate the unmet demand for treatment. These arguments are based on experience with the rapid, large-scale expansion of drug abuse treatment and also on the finding by Watters and colleagues (1986) that nearly half of the out-of-treatment drug users they interviewed said that they would enter treatment "tomorrow" if a position were available.

---

[7] The distinction between publicly funded, non-profit programs and private insurance reimbursed, for-profit programs is not exact. There are some for-profit programs that accept Medicaid insurance, but this is a minority of the for-profit programs, and many persons on waiting lists for publicly funded programs are not Medicaid eligible. The fees at publicly funded programs are much less than those charged by for-profit programs, but can be large enough to discourage many persons with drug abuse problems from even applying for treatment at those programs (Jackson and Rotkiewicz, 1987).

From 1971 through 1974, the New York City Health Department opened 40 methadone maintenance treatment clinics, and more than 22,500 persons were admitted for treatment (Newman, 1977). Applications for treatment were accepted prior to the opening of the clinics (thus creating waiting lists), and the zip code of the applicant's residence was included in the basic information collected in the application, permitting analyses by geographic area. Newman compared the number of new applicants from zip codes that already had methadone clinics (prior to the opening of the Department of Health clinic) with the number of new applicants from zip codes in which the Department of Health clinic was the first in the area (Newman, 1977, p. 110). In the areas with a preexisting clinic, the average number of new applications to the Health Department clinic nevertheless remained relatively constant over time: from 274 in the second month prior to the opening of the Health Department clinic, to 235 in the month immediately preceding opening, to 251 in the month of opening, to 284 in the month after opening, to 231 in the second month after opening. (The clinics provided services to between 250 and 300 patients.) If the waiting list of applications that was established prior to the opening of the clinics had, indeed, represented all of the unmet need for treatment, then there should have been a significant drop in the number of applications after the opening of the clinics. Instead, the number of new applications per month remained relatively constant, suggesting that the opening of the clinic itself brought forth many new applications from persons who would not have applied without the perception that treatment would actually be available.

This potential effect of the perception of treatment availability was even more dramatic in the areas in which there were no preexisting methadone maintenance clinics. In those areas, the number of new applications dramatically increased with the opening of the Health Department clinics: from an average of 279 in the second month preceding opening, to 349 in the month preceding opening, to 706 in the month of opening, to 752 in the month after opening, to 864 in the second month after opening. For these areas without prior methadone treatment, the start of actual provision of treatment was followed by large-scale increases in the number of new applicants. In the light of these results, the preopening waiting list was clearly an underestimate of the actual unmet demand for treatment.

A more recent example involving New York City occurred during the spring of 1988. At that time, the Beth Israel methadone maintenance program had an unduplicated waiting list of approximately 500 persons who had applied but were not currently receiving methadone maintenance treatment. Funds were obtained to add an additional 500 treatment positions to the more than 8,000 treatment positions then in the program. The intent was to reduce or eliminate the waiting list. The 500 new patients were admitted within a period of three months. But only three months later, the waiting list had again stabilized at approximately 500 persons. Hence, the opening of a substantial number of new treatment positions had not led to a permanent reduction in the waiting list but instead brought out new applications from persons who would not have applied without the perception that more treatment was being made available.

The argument that waiting lists underestimate the true unmet demand for treatment can be most easily understood by considering an analogy between waiting lists and the official unemployment rate. Just as waiting lists are composed of persons who are seeking but have not secured treatment, the officially unemployed are persons who are seeking but have not secured employment. Yet in addition to persons who are officially unemployed, there are also "discouraged workers" who might want employment but who have stopped seeking it because they do not expect to be able to find a job. Because they are not actively seeking employment, these discouraged workers are not included in official unemployment calculations. Nevertheless, if large-scale sources of employment develop in their communities, many discouraged workers apply for the positions. Similarly, the opening of new drug treatment positions may lead many persons with drug abuse problems to apply for treatment even though they were not previously on waiting lists.

The analogy between waiting lists and official unemployment figures can be carried at least one step further. If the new jobs are particularly attractive, one would expect larger numbers of discouraged workers to apply for them than might apply for less attractive jobs. So, too, if new treatment programs are particularly attractive, one would expect larger numbers of "discouraged persons with drug problems" to apply for the new treatment positions. Methadone maintenance was a particularly attractive type of treatment for heroin addicts, one that induced many more persons to seek treatment than were on waiting lists prior to its development. A chemotherapy that would both relieve cravings for, and block the effects of, cocaine might be a particularly attractive type of treatment that could attract many more persons than are currently on waiting lists for cocaine treatment.

SHOULD THERE BE WAITING LISTS?

To summarize, some experts believe that current waiting lists accurately reflect unmet demand, others believe that current lists greatly overestimate such demand, and still others believe that current lists greatly underestimate it. Nevertheless, all of these groups tend to agree that the presence of waiting lists is undesirable. There are, however, still other experts in the United States who argue that meaningful waiting lists do exist but that it is desirable to have them.

This argument is not usually presented in terms of the desirability of waiting lists but in opposition to the concept of "treatment on demand." Treatment on demand is not a well-defined term in the drug abuse field; at a minimum, however, it implies a treatment system in which a person would be able to receive treatment immediately after applying. There are two components of the arguments against treatment-on-demand (Kleber, 1990).[8] The first is cost. Kleber has estimated that a true treatment-on-demand system would require that the programs in the system operate at no more than 95 percent of capacity to ensure absorption of any unexpected surge in the number of applications. Estimating the increased costs of operating a drug abuse treatment system in which the programs operated at no more than 95 percent of capacity is beyond the scope of this paper, but it is worthwhile to note that Kleber's formulation could provide a useful empirical standard for assessing unmet demand for treatment independent of the actual number of persons on waiting lists.

Standardized definitions of the capacities of drug abuse treatment programs and of who is enrolled in a treatment program[9] are less than ideal, but clearly they are much easier to formulate than a standardized definition of who is on a waiting list. In addition, the problems of double-counting and transfers do not arise. The factor of perceived treatment availability leading to more new applicants for treatment could also be incorporated into this framework—provided that information about the immediate availability of treatment was disseminated to persons with drug abuse problems. Currently, many programs in the United States operate above 95 percent of capacity (some are operating at above 100 percent of official capacity) so that, by this standard, there is clearly a situation of unmet demand for treatment in the country.

The second argument against treatment on demand concerns the use of waiting lists for motivational screening of applicants. One of the major problems in current forms of drug abuse treatment is the high percentage of persons who drop out of treatment before completion. In addition, up to 50 percent of all applicants never actually enter treatment, and in some types of treatment, up to 50 percent of those who do enter drop out within the first three months (Hubbard et al., 1989; Newman, 1977; Simpson et al., 1978). The long-term effectiveness of treatment in reducing drug abuse— and in reducing HIV risk behaviors (Ball et al., 1988)—is strongly related to the time spent in treatment (Hubbard et al., 1989; Simpson et al., 1978).

---

[8]Kleber is currently the Deputy Director for Demand Reduction of the Office of National Drug Control Policy.

[9]The major difficulty in determining who should be counted as enrolled in a treatment program involves persons who have missed scheduled appointments at the program. After how many missed appointments, or how long after the last missed appointment, should a person still be counted as an enrollee in the program?

Applicants who fail to enter treatment or entrants who drop out shortly after entering represent groups for whom being in treatment provides little or no long-term benefit.

There are undoubtedly many reasons for some applicants' decision not to enter treatment or to drop out so quickly after entering; one frequently cited by clinicians is that these are the people who were never "sufficiently motivated" to actually enter and/or remain in treatment. If being on a waiting list indeed serves to screen out applicants who are not sufficiently motivated to enter and remain in a treatment program, then the waiting list would be serving a positive function by maximizing the effectiveness of scarce drug abuse treatment resources. Consideration of this motivational screening argument leads us to the small number of empirical studies of the behavior of drug users while on waiting lists and the effect on subsequent treatment experience of being on a waiting list.

EMPIRICAL STUDIES OF WAITING LIST BEHAVIOR

As noted earlier, it was quite difficult to find empirical studies of waiting list behavior, and most of the waiting list studies that used controls involved subjects who were already in some form of drug abuse treatment. Moreover, none of the few studies that are directly relevant to the topic of drug user behavior (while not in treatment and on a waiting list) were able to obtain representative samples of the persons on waiting lists at the time. Thus, the limited findings must be interpreted with considerable caution; they do suggest, however, that the topic is quite complex.

Brown and colleagues (1989) conducted a study of 29 persons on a waiting list for a residential treatment program in Baltimore that specialized in treatment of cocaine abuse. The 29 respondents interviewed were recruited from among 50 persons on the waiting list who could actually be contacted, after it was found that less than 50 percent of all persons with whom contact was attempted could actually be reached. Comparisons were made between 16 persons who had been on the waiting list for one to three months, and 13 persons who had been on the waiting list for four to six months. Being on the waiting list for the longer period of time was associated with more criminal justice system involvement and more pressure from others to enter treatment. Forty-eight percent of the total group of subjects had reduced their drug use while on the waiting list, but 59 percent were pessimistic about their ability to remain free of drug use-related problems. Eighty-seven percent of the 23 intravenous drug users in the study reported having changed their behavior to reduce the risk of AIDS, with safer injection as the primary form of risk reduction. A majority of the subjects (52 percent) reported that their interest in entering treatment had decreased since being on the waiting lists. The authors noted that the subjects whom they were able to reach were those who were probably doing relatively well and that any deleterious effects of not being able to enter treatment were probably greater for the waiting list persons whom they were not able to contact.

Patch and colleagues (1973) conducted a study of heroin users who were on a waiting list for methadone maintenance treatment in Boston. The subjects were on the waiting list for periods ranging from 18 months to 2 years. There were high rates of death, incarceration, and family separation among subjects during the time that they were on the waiting lists. The very length of time on the waiting list in this study makes it difficult to draw causal inferences about being on a waiting list and the observed outcomes. Without reapplication to the program or some form of continued contact between the program and subjects, it is not clear what (if anything) being on the waiting list meant to the subjects over such an extended period. This is of particular concern, given the number of studies cited earlier that found that approximately half the persons on waiting lists do not enter treatment when a treatment position opens up and the program attempts to contact them. It is quite possible that, if time on the waiting list had been relatively short (e.g., several weeks to a month), half of the subjects in this study would have been removed from the waiting list without actually entering the program to which they originally applied. Even with this limitation, this study still should be taken as an important caution against allowing long waiting lists to develop.

Gunne and colleagues (Gunne and Gronbladh, 1984) conducted a randomized assignment study of heroin injectors applying for methadone maintenance treatment in Sweden. Thirty-four subjects were randomly assigned to either acceptance into methadone treatment or to a control/no-methadone treatment condition. (The study was ethically justifiable because it would not have been possible to exceed the official capacity of the clinic.) Even though the study involved a small number of subjects, the results were quite dramatic: 76 percent of the treatment group were considered successfully rehabilitated at follow-up versus only 6 percent of the control group. None of the treatment subjects had died, compared with 5 of the 17 control subjects. Because the follow-up period covered more than two years for the subjects, however, this study should be interpreted in terms of denying treatment to persons with heroin addiction problems rather than merely delaying such treatment by putting a person on a waiting list.

Addenbrooke and Rathod (1990) directly examined the relationship between time on a waiting list and later retention in treatment for 130 drug users referred to the Substance Abuse Project at Crawley Hospital, West Sussex, England. The researchers were not testing the motivational screening hypothesis but rather its opposite—that quick entry into treatment would increase motivation and lead to higher retention rates. Ninety of these individuals were accepted for treatment and had a clearly documented date of initial referral. Alcohol use was the primary problem for these individuals, with 69 of the 90 reporting problems associated with alcohol use only. Forty-four of the subjects were accepted into treatment within one week of referral, and 46 were accepted after a longer period. The mean duration of treatment was longer for the quick-entry-into-treatment group (median duration of treatment = 2.9 months) than for those who delayed entry into treatment (median duration of treatment = 1.6 months), but this difference was not statistically significant according to the Mann-Whitney U test. Subjects who had problems with drugs other than alcohol (but no problems with alcohol) stayed in treatment for a shorter period than subjects who had trouble with alcohol only and with alcohol plus other drug use-related problems (medians of 1 and 2.1 months, respectively). In this study, a small number of subjects had problems with drugs other than alcohol, and the relationship between time from referral and retention in treatment was not presented separately for this subgroup. One therefore cannot extrapolate these results to the population of illicit drug users who are the concern of this paper. Clearly, however, the paper does not provide support for the use of waiting lists for motivational screening to increase the cost-effectiveness of drug abuse treatment.

Grenier (1985) conducted a study that used waiting list controls to assess the effectiveness of an adolescent drug abuse treatment program. (Because the persons of interest were minors and because they had not signed informed consent documents, the data were actually collected from their parents.) Only a minority of the persons on the waiting list could be contacted for data collection—27 out of 74—although full cooperation was obtained from all persons who were reached. There was some evidence of improvement among the adolescents on the waiting list. After excluding those who had received other treatment, 14 percent were classified as abstinent from mood-altering drugs and a total of 43 percent as "improved." (The abstinence rate among persons who had received treatment in this particular program was significantly higher—66 percent.) Although this study suggests that the program had a positive influence, the "motivational screening" effect might have undermined the comparison. If the persons who received treatment had to undergo a waiting period prior to entering treatment, there might have been a selection bias toward "more treatment motivation" in this group.

Yancovitz and colleagues (1991) conducted a study of a limited-service "interim" methadone maintenance clinic in New York City. Subjects were recruited from the waiting list of the Beth Israel Medical Center methadone maintenance program and randomly assigned to either immediate entry into the interim clinic or to continuation on the waiting list. Interviews and urinalyses were performed for both groups of subjects.

The study had several limitations. Because the subjects were all volunteers, they cannot be considered a representative sample of persons on the general waiting list for the methadone maintenance program. Moreover, because they were already on a waiting list when they entered the study, any immediate effects of being placed on a waiting list had already occurred for both the experimental and control groups. Yet despite these limitations, this is the only study that could be located that had actual random assignment, multiple time-point follow-up, and urinalysis results. (The study's analyses of self-reported drug use indicated systematic biases.)

At the group level, there was little change in drug use over the one-month follow-up for waiting list controls. Sixty-two percent of the subjects had evidence of heroin use in their urine sample at their entry into the study, and 60 percent had evidence at follow-up. Seventy-one percent had evidence of cocaine use in their urine sample at entry; 70 percent showed such evidence at follow-up. Twenty-six percent had evidence of unprescribed methadone in their urine sample at entry; 37 percent had it at follow-up. This last difference was a statistically significant increase and, given the risk of AIDS when illicit drugs are injected, can be considered some evidence for "improvement" while on the waiting list. (The experimental treatment group showed a highly significant reduction in heroin use and a nonsignificant trend toward a reduction in cocaine use.)

At the individual level, considerable variation occurred over time among the waiting list control subjects. For 26 percent of the subjects, the heroin urinalysis results differed from entry to follow-up. For 31 percent of the subjects, the cocaine urinalysis results differed from entry to follow-up. For 33 percent of the subjects, the methadone urinalysis results differed from entry to follow-up. Although urinalysis detects only recent drug usage (approximately two days for cocaine and one week for heroin and methadone), these results suggest considerable variation over time in drug use by individual subjects in a waiting list condition.

After one month in the waiting list control condition for this study, subjects were then transferred into the interim clinic experimental condition. Eventual enrollment in regular methadone treatment was compared for the group that was immediately assigned to experimental treatment versus the group that remained on a waiting list for an additional month. The subsequent enrollment in regular treatment was significantly higher—72 percent—for the group that had been immediately assigned to treatment than for the group that remained on the waiting list for an additional month—56 percent.

In summary, there are very few studies of the actual behavior of persons on waiting lists. All of these studies have major limitations; in particular, none utilized a representative sample of persons on waiting lists. Nevertheless, these few studies are consistent on several points. First, the behavior of persons on the waiting list is not frozen at the level of behavior observed when the person applied for treatment. There is considerable individual variation over time while subjects are on the waiting list, and the general group direction appears to be toward modest improvement. As expected, the studies that compared being on a waiting list with actually being in drug abuse treatment showed more positive results associated with being in treatment. No evidence could be found that time on a waiting list leads to positive motivational screening in such a way that a longer time waiting would lead to better treatment outcomes for those who do enter treatment. If anything, there is some slight evidence that being placed on a waiting list may have a generally discouraging effect, with a potential net loss of treatment effectiveness.

DISCUSSION

The diversity of expert opinion about waiting lists for drug abuse treatment in the United States is not surprising, given the small amount of empirical research on either the administrative aspects of waiting lists or the behavior of persons while on waiting lists. The discussion in this paper must therefore be a mixture of cautions regarding use of the currently available data and of suggestions for needed additional research.

Current estimates of the number of persons on waiting lists should not be considered accurate quantitative measures of the unmet demand for drug abuse treatment. The unsolved problems of the same individual being on different waiting lists, and of individuals wanting to transfer, in themselves preclude using these estimates as measures of actual unmet demand. Nevertheless, the number of programs that have waiting lists and the number of persons on those lists demonstrate that the present drug abuse treatment system is not effectively meeting the demand for treatment in this country. Some of the unmet demand for treatment could be alleviated by better referral mechanisms among programs. Reviewing studies on the effectiveness of referral systems for drug abuse treatment was beyond the scope of this paper, but caution is necessary here. Referral systems themselves consume scarce resources. Giving a referral to a drug user may satisfy a service provider's need to do something, but it does not even guarantee that the drug user will actually enter that program, much less remain in it. In addition, at a motivational level, drug users may actually do better in programs that they have indicated that they wish to attend, rather than in those that happen to have openings at a given time.

The currently unmeasured number of drug users who desire treatment but do not apply because they do not expect to be taken into treatment needs to be addressed (e.g., Watters et al., 1986). Following the analogy of official unemployment rates, which fail to account for "discouraged" workers, the number of discouraged drug users who would like to enter (but are not seeking) treatment is likely to be greatest when the waiting lists are especially long.

A three-part definition of the desired situation, in which demand for treatment is effectively met, can be proposed:

1. All programs in the system normally operate at 95 percent (or less) of capacity. Capacity is increased for those programs that approach 100 percent utilization.

2. Drug users in the community know that they can be accepted into the treatment program of their choice as soon as they apply.

3. There are no barriers to treatment program entry that would inhibit drug users from applying. Such barriers might include the need for (private or public) health insurance, the need for cash payments, the lack of child care, and the limited treatment modalities available in some cities.

Comparisons of the extent to which different communities are meeting the need for drug abuse treatment would have to include all of these components. Data on the first and third criteria could usually be obtained from program records or interviews with staff, although the latter would preferably also include interviews with users. Data on the second would require interviews with drug users in the community. Fortunately, a number of research projects are currently interviewing large numbers of drug users not in treatment. The National AIDS Demonstration Research studies and the Drug Use Forecasting system could, at very little additional cost, collect data on drug users' perceptions of the availability of treatment.

Finally, given that at present the country appears to be tolerating large (but undetermined) numbers of persons on waiting lists, more research is critically needed on what happens to these drug users. Little is known about the effects of being placed on a waiting list, and almost nothing is known about why so many drug users do not enter treatment when a position becomes available. The new studies should employ better methods than those currently in use. For example, it may not be possible to obtain a perfectly representative sample of persons on a waiting list, but it is surely possible to come much closer to this objective than current studies have done. Larger sample sizes are also necessary to allow examination of the possible differential effects of being on a waiting list, considering such variables as age, gender, ethnicity, and history of drug use.

FINAL COMMENT

In preparing this paper, we have examined opinions and research on waiting lists for drug abuse treatment in the United States. We have conducted research on waiting list behavior and in this paper call for more and better studies on the topic. We also find ourselves deeply troubled by the ethics of performing research on people who need and are awaiting treatment—unless that research is tied to efforts to help them get that treatment. Debating the meaning of waiting lists, without a good faith commitment to provide treatment for all who need it, appears to be even less ethically justifiable.

REFERENCES

Addenbrooke, W. M., and Rathod, N. H. 1990. Relationship between waiting time and retention in treatment amongst substance abusers. *Drug and Alcohol Dependence* 26:255-264.

Ball, J. C., Lange, W. R., Myers, C. P., and Friedman, S. R. 1988. Reducing the risk of AIDS through methadone maintenance treatment. *Journal of Health and Social Behavior* 29:214-226.

Brown, B. S., Hickey, J. E., Chung, A. S., Craig, R. D., et al. 1989. The functioning of individuals on a drug abuse treatment waiting list. *American Journal of Drug and Alcohol Abuse* 15:261-274.

Centers for Disease Control. 1990. Update: Reducing HIV transmission in intravenous drug-users not in drug treatment—United States. *Morbidity and Mortality Weekly Report* 39:529, 535-538.

Des Jarlais, D. C. 1989. AIDS prevention programs for intravenous drug users: Diversity and evolution. *International Review of Psychiatry* 1:101-108.

Friedman, S. R., Neaigus, A., Jose, B., et al. In press. Behavioral outcomes of organizing drug injectors against AIDS. *Proceedings of the Second Annual Research Conference of the National AIDS Demonstration Research Projects*, Rockville, Md.: National Institute on Drug Abuse.

Grenier, C. 1985. Treatment effectiveness in an adolescent chemical dependency treatment program: A quasi-experimental design. *International Journal of the Addictions* 20:381-391.

Gunne, L., and Gronbladh, L. 1984. The Swedish Methadone Program. Pp. 205-213 in *Social and Medical Aspects of Drug Abuse*. G. Serban, ed. New York: Spectrum Publications.

Henik, W., and Domino, G. 1975. Alterations in future time perspective in heroin addicts. *Journal of Clinical Psychology* 31:557-564.

Hubbard, R. L., Marsden, M. E., Rachal, J. V., Harwood, H. J., Cavanaugh, E. R., and Ginzburg, H. M. 1989. *Drug Abuse Treatment: A National Study of Effectiveness*. Chapel Hill and London: University of North Carolina Press.

Ingram, J. A., and Salzberg, H. C. 1990. Effects of in vivo behavioral rehearsal on the learning of assertive behaviors with a substance abusing population. *Addictive Behaviors* 15:189-194.

Institute of Medicine. 1990. *Treating Drug Problems*. D. R. Gerstein and H. J. Harwood, eds. Washington, D.C.: National Academy Press.

Jackson, J., and Rotkiewicz, L. 1987. A Coupon Program: AIDS Education and Drug Treatment. Paper presented at the *Third International Conference on AIDS*, Washington, D.C. , June 4.

Kleber, H. G. 1990. Testimony before the National Commission on AIDS, March 15, 1990.

Korcok, M. 1991. Private addiction treatment faces closings, sell-offs, cuts. *American Medical News*, May 8.

McAuliffe, W. E. 1990. Health care policy issues in the drug abuser treatment field. *Journal of Health and Political Policy Law*, 15:357-385.

Newman, R. G. 1977. Methadone Treatment in Narcotic Addiction. New York: Academic Press.

Patch, V. D., Fisch, A., Levine, M. E., et al. 1973. A mortality study of waiting list patients at the Boston City Hospital methadone maintenance clinic. Pp. 523–529 in *Fifth National Conference on Methadone Treatment Proceedings*. New York.

Presidential Commission on the Human Immunodeficiency Virus Epidemic. 1988. *Final Report of the Presidential Commission on the Human Immunodeficiency Virus Epidemic*. Washington, D.C.: U.S. Government Printing Office.

Simpson, D. D., Savage, L. J., and Sells, S. B. 1978. *Data Book on Drug Treatment Outcomes: Follow-up Study of 1969–1972 Admissions to the Drug Abuse Reporting Program (DARP)*. Report No. 78-10. Fort Worth, Tex.: Institute of Behavior Research, Texas Christian University.

U.S. Conference of Mayors. 1987. *The Anti-Drug Abuse Act of 1986: Its Impact in Cities One Year After Enactment*. Washington, D.C.: The Conference.

U.S. House of Representatives. 1972. *Narcotic Addiction Treatment and Rehabilitation Programs in New York City*. Report to Subcommittee No. 4, Committee on the Judiciary. Washington, D.C.: U.S. House of Representatives.

Watters, J. K., Iura, D. M., and Iura, K. W. 1986. *AIDS Prevention and Education Services to Intravenous Drug Users Through the Midcity Consortium to Combat AIDS: Administrative Report on the First Six Months*. San Francisco: Midcity Consortium.

Yancovitz, S. R., Des Jarlais, D. C., Peyser, N. P., et al. 1991. A randomized trial of an interim methadone maintenance clinic. *American Journal of Public Health* 81:1185-1191.

C

Developing Indicators of Access to Care: The Case for Migrants and the Homeless

Joanne E. Lukomnik [1]

Developing indicators that can monitor progress in ensuring equitable access to health care services is especially difficult when considering some of the most vulnerable populations in the United States. Many of the indicators developed in the main body of this report depend on data reported from national surveys; these data are coded by geographic area and then ascribed to specific communities. Certain population groups, however, are either systematically underrepresented in most national surveys or have other characteristics that make it difficult to track their access to services. Among these populations are migrant farmworkers and their families, the homeless, undocumented workers, and others whose employment or other life circumstances necessitate frequent movement and residential shifts.

This review concentrates on existing knowledge regarding access barriers and the consequent health status of migrant farmworkers and the homeless, two examples of such populations. For these groups, knowledge regarding access to services, barriers to access, and the health consequences of utilization (or the lack of utilization) may depend on our ability to perform periodic special surveys rather than on indicators derived from already existing data bases. This review relies on the sparse published literature as well as program data and experience generated by the Migrant Health (Public Health Service Act, Section 329) and Health Care for the Homeless

[1]Joanne E. Lukomnik is Special Assistant to the Dean, Albert Einstein College of Medicine, the Bronx, New York City, and is also an independent consultant.

(Public Health Service Act, Section 340) programs. The last portion of this paper proposes a series of indicators of barriers to access for these groups and a set of special studies that would provide data on access for these populations that are otherwise lacking today.

The homeless and the migrant farmworker population share a distinctive characteristic in our society: they survive without a permanent home address, a fixed locality where mail can be sent, phones can be installed, and the census bureau can locate them. For example, the National Health Interview Surveys and many studies on access, including the Robert Wood Johnson Foundation (1986) survey on access, rely on telephone contacts to enter respondents into the studies. Such surveys in specific geographic areas frequently also rely on the telephone (e.g., Hubbell et al., 1991). Other surveys use lists of randomly generated household addresses. Because of the lack of a fixed address and the related lack of telephone service, migrant and seasonal farmworkers and the homeless are often excluded from these types of studies. The National Health Interview Survey (NHIS) requires that at least one household member in a respondent household be an English speaker. Because many migrant and seasonal farmworkers are Hispanic or members of recently arrived, non-English-speaking immigrant groups, they may be excluded from the NHIS and other surveys requiring English. Tragically, migrants and the homeless share more than the lack of a fixed address: members of both groups live in extreme poverty, have less than the national average level of education, and have a greater burden of illness, higher rates of infant mortality, and shorter life expectancies than Americans as a whole (National Migrant Resource Program, 1990; Wright and Weber, 1987).

Migrant farmworkers and their families, the single adult living on the street, and homeless families in shelters periodically become "visible." For brief periods, the news media and policymakers focus on the problems of homelessness or the plight of migrants. These news stories include references to the poor health indices of both groups. Despite individual studies and some targeted surveys, however, few systematic national efforts have been made to monitor the health status of members of either group and their access to quality health care. Interestingly, far more is known about the health status and illness patterns of the homeless than about the comparable status of migrants, even though homelessness is only a decade-old phenomenon in its most recent manifestation and migrant farmworkers have been an essential component of agribusiness for more than half a century. Several possible explanations can be postulated. The creation of a class of people known as the homeless was an inadvertent offshoot of other social policies and programmatic decisions. The homeless are highly visible in the nation's cities and media centers, which are also the epicenters of medical and health services research. During the 1980s, as the number of homeless multiplied, attention and new programs proliferated (specifically, the Robert Wood Johnson Foundation's Health Care for the Homeless program and its Public Health Service successor, the McKinney Health Care for the Homeless). In contrast, migrants are seen as a necessary part of the agricultural work force. They are hidden from the view of most people, and their stories seldom capture the attention of the public. Furthermore, there is an assumption that such mechanisms as the migrant health clinics and occupational health and sanitation laws "took care of their problems" long ago. Renewed efforts to improve the health status of migrants and their access to health care services might prove to be quite expensive, requiring reorganization of agricultural labor patterns. These reasons make it easy to postulate a reluctance to focus on migrant health and access issues.

Available information about health status, access to health services, and utilization of the medical system by migrants and seasonal farmworkers and the homeless is generally derived from surveys and evaluations of specially targeted health care delivery systems (e.g., the Migrant Health Clinics and Health Care for the Homeless programs). These studies provide important information, but by definition they are concentrating on that proportion of these populations who have, in fact, gained access, at least briefly, to the medical care delivery system. Because access and utilization cannot be assumed to be synonymous, indicators of access must look beyond utilization figures. Utilization of health care services is a function both of individual attributes of the patient and organizational factors, including the availability and accessibility of health care services. Among individual attributes, the severity of a person's health problem, his or her perception of vulnerability, cultural and psychological attitudes toward physicians and the health care system, and the perceived costs and benefits involved in seeking care will all influence utilization behavior (Aday and Anderson, 1975).

Organizational factors that affect utilization include the economic cost, availability, distance, and location of health care services, appropriate linguistic services, and other economic, ecological, and organizational aspects of the health services themselves (Aday and Anderson, 1984). For the vulnerable populations in question, the homeless and migrant and seasonal farmworkers, measuring access becomes more complicated because the traditional organization of care may fail to meet their individual *or* organizational needs, despite relatively poor health and a documented need for services.

The development of indicators to monitor access to health care services for these populations should be a priority not only in and of itself but also because these groups represent an extreme along a spectrum of vulnerable populations. These populations are known to be at risk for poor health outcomes, which are partially attributable to limited access to appropriate health care services. Although the homeless and migrant populations constitute two groups with known poor health outcomes, they are not, in fact, totally distinct groups. Migrant workers are frequently homeless, particularly between picking seasons. Homeless persons, particularly single men, may enter the migrant stream briefly or intermittently.

More importantly, neither the migrant nor homeless population is stagnant. During the 1980s the nation saw an explosion in the number of poor who found themselves without housing for at least part of the year. Families living in poverty found themselves vulnerable to the threat of homelessness even when they did not experience the actuality. Many people become vulnerable to homelessness through the loss of jobs and income, exhaustion of family support systems, or other tragedies that may precipitate them into homelessness. (Hopper and Hamberg, 1984; U.S. General Accounting Office, 1985). Likewise, the boundary between migrant farmworker, seasonal agricultural worker, and the unemployed often blurs, particularly between agricultural seasons or when bad weather, other natural disasters, or poor economic times limit harvesting of crops. The rural poor may participate in seasonal agricultural work even when not joining the migrant streams.

Although both groups are a heterogeneous population of black, white, Hispanic, Haitian, and other ethnic backgrounds, minorities, who are already at risk for poor health, are disproportionately represented among both the homeless and migrants. Undocumented workers, recent immigrants, and their families often join the migrant streams where few questions about immigration status may be asked. Undocumented workers and recent immigrants may also become homeless because they may not be eligible for welfare or unemployment benefits. Individuals who suffer from mental illness, alcoholism, and drug addiction are represented among the homeless in numbers far exceeding their proportions in the general population (Institute of Medicine, 1988). The living and working environments of migrants may also create or select for individuals with these conditions.

The Institute of Medicine's Committee on Monitoring Access to Personal Health Services defines access as "the timely use of personal health services to achieve the best possible health outcomes." The health care needs of both the migrant and homeless populations are enormous and complex, as a consequence of poverty, environmental and occupational risks, mental health needs, and the living conditions that define and determine the existence of these groups. In turn, monitoring access, evaluating the barriers to health care, and assessing the appropriateness of services for the homeless and for migrant populations are essential to understand the complex relationships among health status, health care utilization, and outcomes. Ultimately, this knowledge must be joined with the political will to guarantee access to high-quality care for these interrelated and most vulnerable of populations.

MIGRANT HEALTH STATUS

Estimates of the number of migrant and seasonal farmworkers and their dependents vary between 2.7 million and 5 million people (National Migrant Resource Program and the Migrant Clinicians Network, 1990). Determining the actual number of migrants is complicated by the number of different federal and state agencies involved in collecting data, the transient nature of the population, systematic undercounting of workers by agribusiness, and the desire of many workers themselves (particularly if they are documented or undocumented immigrants) to avoid contact with any government agencies. The Office of Migrant Health (1992) of the Health Resources and Services Administration quotes a figure of approximately 4 million migrant and seasonal farmworkers and their dependents; this statistic is derived by defining a migrant or seasonal farmworker as "an individual whose principal employment within the last 24 months is in agriculture on a seasonal basis." (Office of Migrant Health, 1992). In this definition, the only difference between a migrant and a seasonal farmworker is that the migrant travels and establishes a temporary abode for employment purposes (Office of Migrant Health, 1992). The Public Health Service divides this number into 1.7 million migrant workers and their dependents and 2.5 million seasonal farmworkers and their dependents. The methodology used to calculate these numbers is complex and includes, in addition to reporting from each state, calculations that estimate the number of person-hours required to harvest the acreage under cultivation.

The Bureau of Labor Statistics uses a narrower definition (employed farmworkers over the age of 14) and notes a steady decline between the 1950s and the early 1980s; it gives a relatively steady current figure of 2.7 million. By this accounting, migrant farmworkers number only 200,000 (not including dependents) with seasonal agricultural workers and other employed farmworkers making up the remaining 2.5 million (U.S. Bureau of the Census, 1990). The Department of Labor and the Department of Agriculture count only employed farmworkers in a given moment in time as reported by employers. Each of these departments uses different methods to calculate the number of employed farmworkers. Neither department estimates the number of dependents or differentiates among farmworkers, crew chiefs, managers, and the like.

All of these estimates are subject to undercounting because of the difficulties inherent in quantifying a work force based on daily hire, the use of crew chiefs who receive the pay for a group of workers, and the still common, although illegal, custom of using children under age 14 (who are excluded from counts by definition) in the fields. The transient and seasonal nature of the work force, and the undocumented movement among Mexico, Central America, Jamaica, and other Latin countries, further complicate the ability to accurately estimate the size of the migrant and seasonal farm-worker population.

The variations and imprecision in population estimates make it extremely difficult to calculate vital statistic rates. A number of sources quote a life expectancy of 49 years, as compared with the national average of 75 years, for migrant farmworkers, and an infant mortality rate that is 125 percent above the national average (National Migrant Resources Program and the Migrant Clinicians Network, 1990). However, literature searches commissioned by the Department of Health and Human Services in 1984, the Farm-worker Justice Fund in 1985 and 1988, and one performed by a migrant health physician in 1990 revealed no published studies that included specific mortality or survival data (Rust, 1990). A literature search performed for this paper and personal communications with personnel from the Office of Migrant Health also failed to discover data on life expectancy, age-specific mortality, or crude death rates.

Recent information about perinatal outcomes is equally hard to obtain. Infant mortality and low-birthweight rates of women using migrant health centers (see the later discussion) have not been calculated. Most studies of birth outcomes are at least 15 years old. In 1978, a study that relied on the mother's recall questioned 132 women in Wisconsin (Slesinger and Christensen, 1986). The authors reported an infant mortality rate of 29 per 1,000 and a mortality rate of 46 per 1,000 children up to the age of 5. Infant mortality among Mexican American farmworkers in Colorado was reported to be 63 per 1,000 in 1971. This rate was three times the national rate for the period (Chase et al., 1971).

The Office of Migrant Health records that 500,000 migrant and seasonal farmworkers and their dependents annually use the 102 migrant health centers located in 43 states and Puerto Rico (These figures are derived from unpublished data for calendar year 1990–1991 from the Health Resources and Services Administration's Bureau of Health Care Delivery and Assistance.) These users represent approximately 17 percent of all migrant and seasonal farmworkers and their families, if one's calculations employ the Public Health Service's number of eligibles as the denominator. We cannot know how representative the users of migrant health centers may be of the total population of migrant and seasonal farmworkers; nevertheless, some information regarding their health status is available and may indicate some general trends.

In a survey of migrant health centers (with a 49 percent response rate from centers representing 54 percent of all patients served nationally), the migrant health centers identified the following as the most common conditions among their maternity and pediatric patients: malnutrition, anemia, hypertension, gestational diabetes, and infection among the pregnant women. For children, the most commonly reported conditions were lack of immunizations, the need for routine exams and dental care, developmental disabilities, dysentery, malnutrition, infectious and parasitic disease, skin disorders, hypertension, fever, measles, and anemia (National Association of Community Health Centers, 1991). Unfortunately, although the list of commonly reported diagnoses is useful, the survey methodology does not permit the calculation of incidence rates.

Another analysis of the migrant health center data used diagnostic codes recorded for all visits during appropriate three-month periods when migrant workers were employed in four migrant centers in three states (Michigan, Indiana, and Texas) that are in the midwestern migratory "stream" (Dever, 1990). The Texan migrant health centers are considered to be "home base" or "downstream" sites, whereas the Indiana and Michigan centers are "non-home base" or "upstream" centers. The study also looked at the demographics of the counties in which the centers were located. The data in the next two paragraphs are drawn from this study (Dever, 1990).

Unfortunately, the study draws conclusions using a mix of data from the counties' demographics and data from the actual encounters at the migrant centers, thereby raising certain methodological questions. Still, the findings indicate an overall trend: using major diagnostic groups (after all the diagnoses were coded according to *International Classification of Diseases*, 9th Revision, Clinical Modification [ICD-9-CM], categories), disorders of the newborn, burns, ear/nose/throat (ENT) conditions, infectious/parasitic disease, injury and poisoning, and eye disorders all exceeded the reported U.S. indices by ranges of from 25 percent to 150 percent. The most common principal diagnoses for all age groups were diabetes mellitus (8.3 percent of total diagnoses), well child care services including immunization (6.7 percent), otitis media (5.9 percent), pregnancy (5.5 percent), upper respiratory infection (4.5 percent), essential hypertension (4.2 percent), contact dermatitis and other eczema (2.5 percent), and hard tissues of the teeth disease (2.2 percent). Beginning with children ages 10–14 and continuing through older age groups, significant dental disease was noted, especially among ages 15–19 for whom hard tissues of the teeth disease accounts for 6.3 percent of all visits, indicating a lack of appropriate dental care at earlier ages. In addition, beginning with adolescence, diseases related to agricultural work begin to appear, especially contact dermatitis, parasitic diseases, sprains and strains, and injury. By late adolescence, ages 15–19, visits for diabetes mellitus begin to be more common. For females in this age bracket, diabetes is the third most common reason (4.6 percent) for seeking care, following only pregnancy and dental disease. Diabetes accounts for an increasing proportion of visits for women throughout all adult age groups. Beginning in their thirties, diabetes becomes an increasingly frequent diagnosis for men. By ages 45–64, the top four diagnoses (diabetes, hypertension, arthropathies, and soft tissue diseases) account for 50 percent of all visits.

When the author of this study compared the top 20 principal diagnoses from the four migrant health centers examined with those reported from the National Ambulatory Medical Care Survey (NAMCS), he found overlap among only 8 diagnostic categories. Twelve of the diagnostic categories noted in data from the migrant health centers did not appear as common visits in the NAMCS data, which represented all U.S. physician visits. These 12 categories included infectious, nutritional, and occupational (including contact dermatitis and eczema) diagnoses. Visits for diabetes were 338 percent above the NAMCS figures. Visits for otitis media and acute respiratory infection were also overrepresented in the migrant health centers (138 percent and 97 percent greater, respectively). As the author correctly notes, using proportions of clinic visits for specific diagnoses fails to provide information regarding disease incidence or prevalence; however, the variation in visits by principal diagnoses between migrants and seasonal farmworkers and their dependents and the general population suggests that migrant and seasonal agricultural workers suffer from different health problems and a greater burden of chronic diseases at a younger age than do most Americans.

Other studies also point to increased health risks among migrant and seasonal farmworkers. Earlier reports documenting the most common diagnoses (at rates far above the national averages) confirm that the major reasons for seeking health care are diabetes, hypertension, and cardiovascular disease. Infectious diseases, especially parasitic diseases, account for a relatively higher proportion of visits than is found among the general population (Health Care Resources, Inc., 1984). The U.S. Bureau of Labor Statistics estimates that there are 12.7 cases of injury and illness per 100 full-time workers per year and 1,700 work-related deaths (52 per 100,000 workers). This makes agriculture the nation's most hazardous occupation. A population-based, cross-sectional study of migrant farmworkers in eastern North Carolina revealed that 8.4 percent (24 of 287 interviewed) had reported an occupational injury during the previous three years (Ciesielski et al., 1991). Another survey reported that 44.5 percent of farmworker households have a disabled individual (InterAmerica Research Association, 1974).

In addition to the injuries and illnesses attributed directly to agricultural work, chronic low-level pesticide exposure carries potential risks, including teratogenesis and carcinogenesis (Rust, 1990). Farmworkers also appear to be at greater risk of acquired immune deficiency syndrome (AIDS) and other infectious diseases, including tuberculosis. A study by the Centers for Disease Control (CDC) in 1988 found a 0.4 percent prevalence of human immunodeficiency virus (HIV) among farmworkers who sought care for any condition; however, a more recent study of farmworkers in the migrant camps of southern New Jersey found a 3.2 percent rate of seropositivity, eight times the national rate (Lyons, 1992).

If knowledge of the health of migrant and seasonal farmworkers and their dependents is limited, an understanding of their health care utilization and the access barriers they actually experience is even more general and inferential. Ninety percent of all migrant families have family incomes below the federal poverty level, and the per-capita income in communities heavily populated by migrant families is half the U.S. average (National Migrant Resource Program, Inc., undated). In 1985, the average migrant farmworker earned only $3,295 per year from farm labor; his or her total income from all sources was only $6,194. (Rust, 1990).

Despite their poverty and the virtual absence of private insurance, migrants and seasonal farmworkers experience more barriers to obtaining Medicaid than other low income groups. A survey of migrant health centers, conducted by the National Association of Community Health Centers in the spring of 1991, documented the remaining barriers, from the providers' perspective, after the Medicaid expansions mandated by Congress in 1989 and 1990 (National Association of Community Health Centers, 1991). Additional barriers to receiving Medicaid benefits would surely emerge if migrants and seasonal farmworkers were queried directly. The survey's most important findings include (1) the difficulty migrants have in establishing state residency and completing the application process before they must move on (these difficulties have persisted despite 1979 Health Care Financing Administration [HCFA] regulations that attempt to ease residency requirements for migrants); (2) the problems migrants experience in retaining coverage and satisfying periodic redeterminations once they receive benefits; (3) the barriers created by documentation and application procedures (because of the time and level of paperwork involved); and (4) the language and cultural barriers inherent in the application process, including the unavailability of forms and translators for non-English-speaking migrants. Forty-three percent of respondents reported mobility-related problems, 43 percent reported language barriers, and 77 percent reported documentation problems. These problems were almost equally present for pregnant women and children—notwithstanding the elimination of categorical eligibility limitations and the liberalization of financial eligibility requirements, which should mean that nearly all pregnant women and children in migrant families would be able to meet Medicaid eligibility standards. Other problems noted by the migrant health centers in this survey included the migrant's inability to comply with face-to-face interview requirements; states' continuing to require permanent residence, despite HCFA guidelines to the contrary; states' denial of benefits to lawful residents because of misapplication of federal alienage standards; and the failure to have hours and locations that are accessible to migrants. These difficulties in obtaining Medicaid benefits were reported by migrant health centers that are presumably highly motivated to help migrants; consequently, the difficulties faced by migrants who are outside the system of migrant health centers can be assumed to be much greater.

Medicaid coverage is only one of the potential factors that enable migrants and seasonal farmworkers to obtain access to necessary health services. A study of health care utilization in Wayne County, New York, performed during the summer of 1982 questioned a sample of migrants living in migrant camps rather than only surveying those utilizing health services (Chi, 1985). This study provides the data in this and the following paragraphs. The study noted that Medicaid recipients, compared with those not receiving Medicaid assistance, had a greater likelihood of visiting physicians for diagnostic and preventive health care. At least in this study, however, factors related to a person's history as a migrant played a more significant role in determining the probability of seeing a physician than did Medicaid status. Migrants who were native born and had been in the migrant stream for a greater length of time were more likely to have seen a physician in the preceding year than were recent immigrants or people new to the migrant stream. Of significance for this study, the county in which this study was conducted contained a federally funded migrant health clinic. Long-term migrants had greater knowledge of, and were more likely to use, this migrant health center. In addition, these long-term migrants were older and slightly better educated, and had a higher probability of having worked in this county or for the same employer previously. Presumably their knowledge of the migrant health center, as well as of the area, increased their ability to navigate through the health care system and gain access to care. Of those migrants who were recent immigrants, 45 percent had no knowledge of the migrant health center, as compared with only 10.4 percent of the long-term migrants. Fifty-one percent of the recent-immigrant migrants had not seen a physician in the preceding year. For all migrants, 64 percent had not seen a physician or had only seen a physician once during the previous year, a far smaller figure than the national norm. As with the general population, female migrants saw physicians more frequently than male migrants.

Equally of interest, more than 40 percent of migrant farm workers in the sample delayed medical care or treatment for an existing medical or dental problem including such conditions as anemia, arthritis, blood in stools, hypertension, broken bones, ulcers, and chest pain. Migrants cited lack of time, followed by economic cost and lack of access (nonspecific), as the reasons cited for delaying care. Almost 25 percent listed fear or lack of confidence in the medical profession as a reason for not seeking or delaying care.

In the population-based study of occupational injuries among North Carolina migrant farmworkers conducted by Ciesielski and colleagues (1991), 11 of the 17 more seriously injured workers (65 percent) either did not receive prompt care (7/17, or 41 percent) or never received care at all (4/17, or 24 percent). Injured farmworkers who did not receive prompt care were twice as likely to have incomplete recoveries. Refusal by the crew leader to allow workers to seek care and lack of transportation prevented 24 percent from receiving care within 24 hours and 42 percent from keeping follow-up appointments. Although this study focused on occupational injuries, an incidental finding was that 19.6 percent of the farmworkers who worked in the tobacco fields of North Carolina reported nausea, and 18.6 percent reported dizziness. None of the farmworkers reported these symptoms as injury.

Studies such as these, which survey migrants directly, can add a great deal to our knowledge of migrant health care utilization behavior and the barriers to access faced by migrants. Combined with information about self-perceived health status and health practices, these studies would allow for appropriate measures of access, as well as provide important information about disease incidence and prevalence. Unfortunately, a literature search failed to turn up additional studies of this kind.

HEALTH STATUS OF THE HOMELESS

As with migrants, there is no consensus on the number of homeless people in this country. The inability to agree on this number (the denominator) makes calculations of rates of disease and health-related problems, as well as measures of access, extremely problematic. Many observers consider the federal estimate derived from the 1990 census, 228,621, too low; these observers include local and state government officials, advocates—and even the Census Bureau itself (*Noah*, 1991). Estimates of the homeless population vary from this low census number to several million. According to the *Wall Street Journal*, in 1989 the Urban Institute estimated the homeless population at 600,000; yet estimates of homeless youths alone, age 21 and younger, from the National Network for Runaway and Homeless Youth, range from 250,000 to several million. The number of homeless families, of mentally ill homeless, of rural homeless, and of homeless elderly are also in dispute.

Despite this inability to quantify the extent of homelessness, an enormous number of studies of the health care needs and health status of homeless people have been published since homelessness emerged as a major national policy issue in the early 1980s. Pioneering work on delivering health care to the homeless and studying their health problems was done under the direction of Philip Brickner, M.D., at St. Vincent's Hospital in New York City (Brickner et al., 1990). In 1985, the Robert Wood Johnson Foundation, the Pew Memorial Trust, and the United States Conference of Mayors established Health Care for the Homeless Demonstration Projects in 19 large cities. (Wright and Weber, 1987). All of the Health Care for the

Homeless projects funded through this program participated in a major research effort directed by the University of Massachusetts' Social and Demographic Research Institute. In addition, a number of surveys and special studies have focused on the relationship between homelessness and mental illness (Blackwell et al., 1990) and homelessness and alcohol and substance abuse (Institute of Medicine, 1988).

Reviews of these studies reveal that the homeless suffer from many of the same acute and chronic illnesses that afflict people in the general population but at much higher rates (Brickner et al., 1990). Because the homeless have little or no access to adequate bathing and hygienic facilities, survive on the streets or in unsafe and generally unsanitary shelters, smoke and drink to excess, and suffer from inadequate diets, their physical health is compromised. Among the findings from the Health Care for the Homeless Demonstration Projects were that the most commonly reported acute conditions were upper respiratory infections, trauma, and skin ailments. Nutritional deficiencies were found in 2 percent of those seen. Of patients seen more than once, 37 percent had at least one chronic condition including hypertension, arthritis and other musculoskeletal disorders, dental problems, gastrointestinal and neurological disorders, peripheral vascular disease, genitourinary problems, and chronic obstructive pulmonary disease. The use of estimation techniques based on recorded diagnoses led to estimates that 38 percent of the homeless seen in the demonstration projects abused alcohol, 13 percent abused drugs other than alcohol, and 33 percent were mentally ill. During the demonstration period, the rates of tuberculosis (968 cases/100,000 population) and AIDS (230 cases/100,000) were significantly higher than those of the general population (e.g., 9 cases/100,000 for TB) (Wright and Weber, 1987). While these findings reflect the homeless population that sought care from the demonstration projects, which may inflate the burden of illness, the demographic characteristics of the patients seen in the demonstration projects did not differ significantly from those described in many ethnographic studies of the homeless (Wright and Weber, 1987).

As with the migrant and seasonal farmworker population, it is difficult to calculate vital statistic rates for the homeless. Not only is the denominator in dispute, but neither birth nor death statistics record homelessness. A study conducted in New York City compared infants born to women living in welfare hotels with infants born to women living in low-income housing projects. The babies born to homeless women living in the hotels were more likely to be of low birthweight (18 percent vs. 8.5 percent) and had a higher infant mortality rate (Chavkin et al., 1987). At the other end of the age spectrum, many who work with the homeless report that very few are over the age of 55, which suggests that the homeless die young. In support of this contention, the median age of those seen in the Health Care for the

Homeless Demonstration program was 33 (Knight and Lam, 1986). A 1984 study of Baltimore's homeless found that only 2 percent were age 65 or older, compared with 18.1 percent of the general population (O'Connell et al., 1990).

It is always difficult to disentangle the effects of access to health care, or, conversely, lack of access, on health status; for the homeless, the difficulties in doing so increase exponentially. Indeed, poor health and the resulting inability to work, often byproducts of homelessness, may also result in homelessness. Although homeless people may have the same array of acute and chronic problems as one finds in the general population, the rates are clearly higher, and the numbers of comorbidities, including alcohol/substance abuse and mental illness, are far in excess of these rates for the general population. Many of these conditions and morbidities are amenable to medical intervention; routine health care should prevent some diseases altogether and minimize exacerbations and complications of chronic diseases. Yet the personal health care services needed by the homeless may require a different organizational configuration, a different array of services, and a different mix of providers than those required for the domiciled population. These suppositions, as well as the inability of traditional clinics and hospitals to care for the homeless adequately, gave rise to the Health Care for the Homeless Demonstration Projects and the subsequent U.S. Public Health Service's McKinney Health Care for the Homeless Program. These demonstrations rely on community-based programs that are often colocated in places in which the homeless may be found in large numbers, such as congruent feeding programs and shelters.

Although the evidence that the homeless lack access to health services, except through targeted programs, is anecdotal and inferential, it is quite convincing. In the 1988 Institute of Medicine report *Homelessness, Health, and Human Needs* the chapter on access reviews the limitations in systems of care for the poor and medically indigent (e.g., in public general hospitals and not-for-profit hospitals serving the poor, clinics, the National Health Service Corps, categorical programs, mental health and Veterans Administration systems, and Medicaid programs) and suggests that, in general, the homeless compete with the poor for these services. In addition to general underfinancing of health care services for the poor, the report identified additional barriers to access facing the homeless: bureaucratic and scheduling issues, lack of transportation, negative perceptions on the part of providers and institutions, and the avoidance of institutions by the homeless themselves because of prior experience (Institute of Medicine, 1988). Despite the lack of quantifiable data, no one has disputed the statements made on the original brochure for the Health Care for the Homeless Demonstration Projects: "Most homeless people do not now receive needed health services. Many are afraid of large institutions, most are uninsured, and many are perceived in some sense to be 'undesirable' as patients" (Robert Wood Johnson Foundation, 1983).

Local coalitions have attempted to document the lack of health care received by the homeless, generally by interviewing patients during a health care visit. In St. Louis, for example, reports indicate that, of the homeless seeking care, more than 70 percent had no usual health care provider and more than half had not received any health care attention in the previous year (Wright and Weber, 1987). In the study of pregnant homeless women living in New York City's welfare hotels (Chavkin et al., 1987), 56.4 percent of the women from the hotels reported three or fewer prenatal visits, compared with 22.5 percent of women in low-income housing projects and 15 percent of women citywide. The New York Children's Health Project reported that in calendar year 1988, of the 3,084 children seen, only 52 percent were adequately immunized and many were undertreated for acute and chronic illnesses. Both findings were attributed to poor or no access to health care services (Brickner et al., 1990).

Few systematic or rigorous studies have been done at shelters, on the streets, or at other gathering places. As discussed earlier, surveys on access generally rely on telephone interviews, thereby eliminating the possibility of participation by the homeless. The general agreement among policymakers and advocates that the homeless continue to have inadequate access to appropriate health care services has not been tested. Because no new federal money has been available for the McKinney Health Care for the Homeless program, few cities or rural areas have performed recent systematic health care needs assessments of this population group. Many cities and advocacy groups do report that the number of homeless continues to increase, which in turn suggests that additional service capacity is needed.

RECOMMENDATIONS

For two of the most vulnerable populations in this country—migrants and seasonal farmworkers and their families, and the men, women, and children who are homeless—neither the traditional measures of access nor the IOM committee's recommended indicators will provide the necessary information to measure and analyze either the barriers that prevent these groups from receiving appropriate, high-quality health care or the nation's progress toward ensuring equity of access. Despite some increased knowledge about the health status and health care needs of both the migrant and homeless populations (with considerably more information about the homeless), we still lack certain baseline measures regarding the access and health care needs of both populations. Although this paper is meant to discuss the development of indicators of access for these populations, indicators of access must include an assessment of unmet health care needs. Information regarding resource allocation and effectiveness is necessary as well.

Neither the migrant/seasonal farmworkers nor the homeless are homogeneous populations. Both groups are made up of various subgroups. The health care needs and access experiences of a Chicano migrant family in the Texas Rio Grande valley will be very different from those of a single man in the East Coast migrant stream. The health care needs of a mentally ill homeless woman on the streets of New York City and her ability to maneuver through the health care system differ enormously from those of a family living in a shelter or of a young displaced worker in a rural area. Much more information is needed to understand the differing health care needs of these subgroups.

Most importantly, our need for information cannot be divorced from our commitment to provide many different types of services to these populations. The IOM study on access is limited in its scope to access to personal health care services. Yet, for migrants and the homeless, the most significant access issues involve access to social, environmental, and occupational reforms that will promote health and prevent disease, as well as to personal health care services. Tracking programs designed to eliminate homelessness must accompany monitoring of the access of homeless people to health care services. Monitoring access to health care services for migrants is good health policy only if we also document migrants' access to safe drinking water and decent living conditions. We seek information from indicators of access to inform health care policy. For the migrants and the homeless, monitoring access to personal health care services is a necessary but insufficient step in understanding the interacting factors that contribute to excess morbidity and mortality in these populations.

The following recommendations address some of the gaps in our knowledge regarding access.

• **The Migrant Health programs (Section 329 of the Public Health Service Act) and the McKinney Health Care for the Homeless programs (Section 340 of the act) should develop data systems that include clinical information necessary to assess the health status of these populations and information regarding utilization of health care services and access barriers encountered within the health care system.** Although this information will come from those migrants and homeless people who already use the two components of the health care system that have been specifically designed to minimize access barriers, much useful information can be collected, as seen by the studies done for the original Health Care for the Homeless Demonstration Projects (Wright and Weber, 1987). Particularly because both migrants and the homeless are relatively mobile populations, their experiences in obtaining health care will vary over time and by location. Surveys of patients using Migrant Health Centers and Health Care for the Homeless programs at one point in time may provide information about their experiences in accessing other services.

Unfortunately, with the conversion of support of Health Care for the Homeless programs from foundations to the Public Health Service, neither the funding nor the commitment to maintaining this complicated information base on the homeless continued. The Bureau of Health Care Delivery and Assistance (BHCDA) of the Health Resources and Services Administration (HRSA), the agency that oversees these programs, has recently committed itself to developing a system for collecting demographic and clinical information. The necessary fiscal and personnel support must be guaranteed to ensure that the data collected provide the information needed on the health status, utilization patterns, and access issues faced by these two populations. The data collected by the BHCDA must therefore include the findings from systematic health evaluations as well as the problems individuals present in seeking help at an appointment. Longitudinal information should be sought whenever possible.

• **Because most indicators are derived from secondary sources or telephone/household surveys in which both migrants and the homeless are underrepresented, special, community-based surveys should be developed to provide information about health status and access.** These surveys should be carried out in migrant camps, homeless shelters, congruent feeding facilities, and other such locations to gain a more complete picture than is currently available. In addition, sampling techniques need to be developed to ensure adequate representation of the subgroups that make up these populations. Surveys also need to be conducted in multiple geographic regions of the country to capture regional differences. The surveys should be patterned after the National Health Interview Survey, the National Health and Nutritional Evaluation, and the Robert Wood Johnson Foundation Access Survey in order to permit national comparisons. Supplemental questions should be developed to address the special circumstances of migrants and the homeless.

• **In coordination with the development of these surveys, the Federal Interagency Committee on Migrants (which is convened quarterly by the Office of Migrant Health and includes representatives from the Departments of Education, Justice, Labor, and Agriculture, and from the Environmental Protection Agency) should develop a research agenda on migrant health issues that would include specific measures of access to personal health care services, including alcohol and substance abuse treatment and mental care health programs.** In addition to the measures of access to these services, the research agenda must include studies that allow for calculating vital statistic rates including maternal and infant mortality, low birthweight, and age- and cause-specific mortality.

Special studies may be needed to establish rates of hospitalization for "ambulatory-sensitive conditions" in order to develop comparisons.

The Federal Interagency Committee on Migrants should be expanded to include representatives from state and local government and advocacy groups (e.g., the National Governors Association, the Association of State and Territorial Health Officers, the National Association of Community Health Centers, the Migrant Clinicians' Network).

• **The Health Care for the Homeless program should initiate a similar interagency group on the homeless. One of the immediate tasks of such a group would be the development of a research agenda.** Many of the same topics, especially the need for information regarding access and the need for vital statistics, are as relevant to the homeless as they are to migrants. Additional issues related to access particularly for the homeless, include the relationships among poor health status (especially mental health), lack of access to appropriate health care services, and the precipitation or continuation of homelessness.

• **Special studies should be undertaken to evaluate the effectiveness of targeted initiatives in increasing access.** These initiatives include, for example, changes in Medicaid and Supplemental Security Income (SSI) eligibility requirements (including guidelines for presumptive eligibility), outstationing of enrollment workers, and changes in residency requirements.** Many of these initiatives were specifically designed to make enrollment and retention of Medicaid benefits easier for migrants and homeless people. Whether these initiatives have succeeded remains to be evaluated.

• **Special studies are needed to examine nonfinancial barriers to care, especially provider and institutional willingness to provide services to these populations, the influence of organizational structure and hours of service on accessibility, transportation and translation services, and other factors that might influence the willingness of patients to seek services.** Both the migrant and homeless populations, or some subgroups among them, may also experience nonfinancial barriers that differ in kind or in scope from those experienced by other population groups.

• **The feasibility of designing special coding for hospital discharges and birth and death certificates to identify the homeless and migrants should be explored.** Although this plan may not prove to be feasible or cost-effective nationally, a targeted study in certain regions might provide important information now lacking.

• **National surveys and followback studies (for example, the National Center for Health Statistics' Mortality Followback survey) should specifically ask whether the index case, or any family member covered by the survey, was ever homeless or ever worked as a migrant.** Occupation is surveyed in some studies, but the question is generally asked in relationship to work in the two weeks prior to administration of the survey; this restriction may lead to a failure to identify migrants and seasonal farm-workers. Household address is almost always requested, yet information may be lacking to indicate whether the address represents a shelter or temporary housing. Although these surveys probably do not sample enough migrants or homeless to allow for subgroup analysis, the information may prove useful, depending on the extent of the response.

• HRSA has cooperative agreements with most state departments of health and supports primary care associations in many states. **In developing primary care needs assessments, state departments of health should be encouraged to develop specific assessments of needs and resources for migrant and the homeless, complete with estimations of the number of individuals affected in each local geographic area.** Qualitative data, including interviews with care providers, local health care institutions, and advocates and representatives of the homeless and migrants, should be included to assess the accessibility of existing services.

• Many state and local health departments have developed infant mortality reviews to ascertain contributing factors. **Infant mortality reviews should specifically address whether the infant in question was homeless or the child of migrants.** The information gleaned from infant mortality reviews should be aggregated nationally for many purposes. With this kind of aggregation, the deaths of migrant and homeless infants could be analyzed as a separate subgroup.

Unfortunately, developing indicators for monitoring the access to health care services of migrants and the homeless cannot be divorced from the need for special studies. There exists a national commitment to providing targeted services through the McKinney Health Care for the Homeless and the Migrant Health Center programs. These programs, however, have had only small increases in funding (less than is necessary to keep up with inflation in the health sector), and few would argue that they have solved the access problems of the majority of migrants or homeless people. If we are to understand the remaining barriers and the extent to which limitations in access contribute to the reported poor health of both groups, we must commit sufficient resources to perform the necessary studies.

REFERENCES

Aday, L. A. and Anderson, R. M. 1975. *Development of Indices of Access to Medical Care.* Ann Arbor, Mich.: Health Adventist Press.

Aday, L. A. and Anderson, R. M. 1984. The national profile of access to medical care: Where do we stand? *American Journal of Public Health* 74:1331.

Blackwell, B., et al. 1990. Psychiatric and mental health services. Pp. 184-203 in Brickner, P. W., Scharer, L. K. et al., eds. 1990. *Under the Safety Net: The Health and Social Welfare of the Homeless in the United States.* New York: Norton.

Brickner, P. W., Scharer, L. K. et al., eds. 1990. *Under the Safety Net: The Health and Social Welfare of the Homeless in the United States.* New York: Norton.

Chase, H. P., Kumar, V., Dodds, J. M., Sauberlich, H. E., et al. 1971. Nutritional status of preschool Mexican-American migrant farm children. *American Journal of Diseases of Children* 122:316-324.

Chavkin, W., Kristal, A., Seaborn, C., and Guigli, P. 1987. The reproductive experience of women living in hotels for the homeless in New York City. *New York State Journal of Medicine* 87:10-13.

Chi, P. 1985. Medical utilization patterns of migrant farm workers on Wayne County, New York. *Public Health Reports* 100:480-490.

Ciesielski, S., Hall, P. and M. Sweeney. 1991. Occupational injuries among North Carolina migrant farmworkers. *American Journal of Public Health* 81:926-927.

Dever, A. 1990. *Migrant Health Status: Profile of a Population with Complex Health Problems.* Austin, Tex: Migrant Clinicians Network Monograph Series.

Health Care Resources, Inc. 1984. An Assessment of Selected Health Conditions of Migrant and Seasonal Farmworkers: Draft Report on the Literature Search. Prepared for the Bureau of Health Care Delivery and Assistance, Health Resources and Services Administration, Washington, D.C.

Hopper, K., and J. Hamberg. 1984. *The Making of America's Homeless: From Skid Row to the New Poor, 1945–1984.* Working Papers in Social Policy. New York: Community Service Society.

Hubbell, F. A., Waitzkin, H., Mishra, S. I., Dombrink, J., and Chavez, L. R. 1991. Access to medical care for documented and undocumented Latinos in a southern California county. *Western Journal of Medicine* 154:414-417, April.

Institute of Medicine. 1988. *Homelessness, Health and Human Needs.* Washington, D.C.: National Academy Press.

InterAmerica Research Association. 1974. *Handicapped Migrant Farmworkers.* U.S. Department of Health, Education, and Welfare Pub. OHD 75-25084. Washington, D.C.: U.S. Government Printing Office.

Knight, J. W., and Lam, J. 1986. *Homelessness and Health: A Review of the Literature.* Amherst, Mass.: SADRI.

Migrant Health Newsline. 1992. Vol. 9, No. 2. Austin, Tex.: National Migrant Resource Program.

National Association of Community Health Centers. 1991. *Medicaid and Migrant Farmworker Families: Analysis of Barriers and Recommendations for Change.* Washington, D.C.: NACHC.

National Migrant Resource Program. Undated. *A Migrant Health Status: Profile of a Culture with Complex Health Problems.* Austin, Tex.: The Program.

National Migrant Resource Program and the Migrant Clinicians Network. 1990. *Migrant and Seasonal Farmworker Health Objectives for the Year 2000.* Austin, Tex.: The Program.

Noah, T. 1991. Census Bureau's count of homeless fails to end debate. *Wall Street Journal* April 15, p. B5C.

O'Connell, J., Summerfield, J. and R. Kellogg. 1990. The homeless elderly. P. 151-153 in Brickner, P. W., Scharer, L. K. et al., eds. 1990. *Under the Safety Net: The Health and Social Welfare of the Homeless in the United States.* New York: Norton.

Office of Migrant Health, Health Resources and Services Administration. 1992. *Farmworker Health for the Year 2000: 1992 Recommendations of the National Advisory Council on Migrant Health.* Rockville, Md.: U.S. Department of Health and Human Services.

Robert Wood Johnson Foundation. 1983. Health Care for the Homeless Program. Princeton, N.J.: The Foundation.

Robert Wood Johnson Foundation. 1986. *Access to Health Care in the United States: Results of 1986 Survey.* Special Report 2, Princeton, N.J.: The Foundation.

Rust, G. 1990. Health status of migrant farmworkers: A literature review and commentary. *American Journal of Public Health* 80:1213-1217.

Slesinger, D., and B. Christensen. 1986. Health and mortality of migrant farm children. *Social Science and Medicine* 23:65-74.

U.S. Bureau of the Census. 1990. *Statistical Abstract of the United States.* 110 Ed. Washington, D.C.: U.S. Department of Commerce, pp. 636-64.

U.S. General Accounting Office. 1985. *Homelessness: A Complex Problem and the Federal Response.* Washington, D.C.: U.S. Government Printing Office.

Wright, J. D., and Weber, E. 1987. *Homelessness and Health.* Washington, D.C.: McGraw-Hill.

D

"Ambulatory-Care-Sensitive" Conditions and "Referral-Sensitive" Surgeries

"AMBULATORY-CARE-SENSITIVE" CONDITIONS

Condition and ICD-9-CM Code(s)	Comments
Congenital Syphilis [090]	Secondary diagnosis for newborns only
Immunization-related and preventable conditions [033, 037, 045, 320.0, 390, 391]	Hemophilus meningitis [320.2] age 1–5 only
Grand mal status and other epileptic convulsions [345]	
Convulsions "A" [780.3]	Age 0–5
Convulsions "B" [780.3]	Age >5
Severe ENT infections [382, 462, 463, 465, 472.1]	Exclude otitis media cases [382] with myringotomy with insertion of tube [20.01]

Chronic obstructive pulmonary disease
[491, 492, 494, 496, 466.0]

Acute bronchitis
[466.0] only with
secondary diagnosis of
491, 492, 494, 496

Bacterial pneumonia [481, 482.2, 482.3,
482.9, 483, 485, 486]

Exclude case with
secondary diagnosis of
sickle cell [282.6] and
patients <2 months

Asthma [493]

Congestive heart failure [428, 402.01,
402.11, 402.91, 518.4]

Exclude cases with
the following surgical
procedures: 36.01,
36.02, 36.05, 36.1, 37.5,
or 37.7

Hypertension [401.0, 401.9, 402.00,
402.10, 402.90]

Exclude cases with
the following
procedures: 36.01,
36.02, 36.05, 36.1, 37.5,
or 37.7

Angina [411.1, 411.8, 413]

Exclude cases with a
surgical procedure
[01-86.99]

Cellulitis [681, 682, 683, 686]

Exclude cases with a
surgical procedure [01-
86.99], except incision
of skin and subcu-
taneous tissue [86.0]
where it is the only
listed surgical procedure

Skin grafts with cellulitis
[DRG 263, DRG 264]

Exclude admissions
from SNF/ICF

Diabetes "A" [250.1, 250.2, 250.3]

Diabetes "B" [250.8, 250.9]

Diabetes "C" [250.0]

Hypoglycemia [251.2]

Gastroenteritis [558.9]

Kidney/urinary infection
[590, 599.0, 599.9]

Dehydration—volume depletion [276.5]   Examine principal
                                            and secondary diagnoses
                                            separately

Dental Conditions [521, 522, 523, 525, 528]

"REFERRAL-SENSITIVE" SURGERIES

Condition and ICD-9-CM Code(s)	Comments
Hip/joint replacement [81.41, 81.48, 81.5, 81.6]	
Breast reconstruction after mastectomy [85.7, 85.95]	Women only
Pacemaker insertion [37.7]	
Coronary artery bypass surgery [36.1]	
Coronary angioplasty [36.01, 36.02, 36.05]	

Index